WHO CARES?

Also by Anthony C. Gatrell and published by Agenda

Global Health: Geographical Connections

WHO CARES?

The Unequal Geographies of Healthcare

ANTHONY C. GATRELL

agenda
publishing

Agenda Publishing is an imprint of Edinburgh University Press, one of the leading university presses in the UK. Publishing new research in the arts and humanities, EUP connects people and ideas to inspire creative thinking, open new perspectives and shape the world we live in. For more information, visit www.edinburghuniversitypress.com.

Edinburgh University Press Ltd
13 Infirmary Street, Edinburgh EH1 1LT

ISBN 978-1-78821-919-8 (hardcover)
ISBN 978-1-78821-920-4 (paperback)

A CIP record for this book is available from the British Library

Typeset by Newgen Publishing UK
Printed and bound in the UK using 100% renewable electricity by CPI Group (UK) Ltd.

EU Authorised Representative:
Easy Access System Europe
Mustamäe tee 50, 10621 Tallinn, Estonia
gpsr.requests@easproject.com

CONTENTS

PREFACE

In 1936 the American political scientist Harold Lasswell published a book on politics whose focus was: "who gets what, when, how". Geographers like me want to add "where" to the subject, since services – of whatever type – have to be delivered some*where*.

The focus of this book is healthcare services. Where people live can dictate what access they have to those (diverse) services that provide healthcare. The aim of this book is to use a geographical imagination to illuminate key issues relating to "access" to (both provision and use of) healthcare services, whether at global, national or local scales. It seeks both to provide a rich body of evidence concerning the unequal production and consumption of such care, and to offer explanations of such disparities. Its key focus is what a geographical imagination can bring to our understanding of the determinants and nature of healthcare: *what difference, and why, does place make?* It is over 40 years since Alun Joseph and David Phillips wrote a key text on this subject: *Accessibility and Utilization: Geographical Perspectives on Health Care Delivery.* The time is ripe for a new look at the subject, not least because of international and national changes to healthcare systems, whether shaped by neoliberalist agendas, disruptive world leaders or new technologies.

I choose to consider the unequal geographies of healthcare and not the geography of health inequalities since there are many books and articles that address geographic variations in health outcomes, and the inequalities that these variations reveal. Among the reasons for these geographic variations are social and economic conditions and we need a good grasp of the political economy of health to understand these. The literature on health inequalities suggests that access to healthcare plays a rather limited role in contributing to health inequalities. But, clearly, if there is a long wait for a consultation or surgery then conditions may well deteriorate for the individual, resulting in poorer outcomes or even premature mortality. These waiting times are, as we shall see, socially patterned, with better-off people able to afford private healthcare that others cannot.

The availability and use of healthcare services is therefore a topic of considerable public interest and concern. Why can I not get to see my family doctor soon? Why am I waiting so long for my operation? How do people get to the clinic or hospital, a journey that looks very different if living in a resource-poor part of the world? Why, and where, are there delays in accessing mental health services? What role (actual and potential) do new technologies play in delivering healthcare? The introductory chapter gives some specific examples of these sorts of issues, and confirms that these issues are not restricted to one country or one healthcare system. They are universal concerns.

I chose the title carefully to show that my focus is mostly on access to "services" that maintain or improve health. What this means is that the book deals mainly with primary and secondary (hospital-based) care services. While the cultural geographies of care (more broadly) are not the focus I address these where appropriate. The book is not "just" about medical care.

In writing this book I have had support from a number of people. Camilla Erskine, formerly of Agenda Publishing, commissioned and encouraged the work. Steven Gerrard at Agenda Publishing has been a great support, while Gillian Bourn was a wonderful copy editor. I am grateful to Clare Owen, Production Editor at Newgen, for her considerable help at the proof-checking stage. Two readers of the manuscript offered careful and constructive comments on the manuscript and I thank them warmly for their generosity. My immediate family – Caroline, Anna and Emma – have followed the book's progress and their love and support continues to mean a great deal.

When I wrote my first book, over 40 years ago, I thanked the various teachers, both at high school and university, from whom I learnt so much. One of my most influential mentors, Peter Haggett, died as the book was nearing completion. As a distinguished medical/health geographer, and much else besides, his influence has remained with me, not only through his scholarship and teaching but also through his *care* as a human being.

Tony Gatrell
Lancaster

LIST OF FIGURES, TABLES AND BOXES

Figures

Tables

Boxes

1 INTRODUCTION

I want to begin by telling four stories about experiences of healthcare.

In 2021 Wendy Davey was living with her husband Derek in a village in north Somerset, in the south-west of England. They were about 30 miles away from their nearest hospital. Wendy, in her late 70s, had suffered a stroke early in 2021 but in October that year she woke in the night with severe trembling in her legs, followed by convulsions and subsequent slurring of speech. Derek called for an ambulance, thinking she was having another stroke.

The National Health Service (NHS) in England sets a standard for ambulance (emergency) response times in the case of suspected heart attacks or stroke; the target is that an ambulance should arrive within 18 minutes. The ambulance that Derek called for took three hours to arrive. "Terrified, I was absolutely terrified," Wendy said, telling her husband she feared she was about to die.

Wendy survived but has needed physiotherapy to help her walk again. Getting appointments for such therapy provided by the NHS proved difficult so she decided to pay for private treatment. That cost her almost £10,000. "If I didn't have any savings, I don't know how I would have survived," Davey said. "It would have been a case of just sitting in a chair with somebody coming in and washing me and getting me dressed. I would be just useless".[1]

Healthcare for Wendy was a matter of her age and infirmity. It was also a matter for her husband Derek. It is a matter too for the healthcare system that has to fund her care. Looking after Wendy depended initially on the geography of provision: where an ambulance was located in relation to where she lived. But accessing subsequent care proved challenging, so she decided to pay for more timely treatment. Not everyone can afford that. For Wendy, healthcare was a matter of both where she lived and her ability to pay to circumvent a lengthy waiting list for subsequent treatment.

Nurse Sadia Khan works at a health centre in Nangarhar Province, in the eastern region of Afghanistan. She lives an hour away from the health centre (reminding us that

1. www.bloomberg.com/graphics/2023-nhs-missing-targets-on-75th-anniversary/

proximity applies to healthcare workers as well as those, like Wendy, seeking care) and worries about not being able to work. The restriction on women's rights in Afghanistan is well-known. "I pray that the Taliban don't stop me from going to work. We [health workers] are exempt from the ban, but I am always apprehensive about the possibility of being stopped by the Taliban and sent home". She also worries about her ability to provide care that is needed:

> A few weeks ago, a woman visited the health centre with a diabetic foot infection. We referred her to a provincial hospital, but she was unable to afford the transportation charges to go to the city. The woman returned the next day, hoping that I would be able to treat her. Unfortunately, there was little that could be done for her at our health centre. It breaks my heart when I see patients who can't get the medical care they need due to financial constraints.[2]

What we take from this story is that accessing care depends on both a patient's needs and how easy it is (here, in terms of distance) for them to get treated. But it also depends on having a healthcare professional being available and how easy it is, or not, for that person themselves to get to a clinic. Travel for Sadia is not merely a matter of distance, but of danger too. Getting looked after by nurse Sadia (Figure 1.1) involves what some geographers would call an "assemblage": a network of actors comprising people, clinics, medicines, transport and so on (Gatrell 2023: 9).

Brian Sinclair was a 45-year-old Indigenous man who lived in Manitoba, Canada and was admitted to the emergency department in the provincial capital, Winnipeg, in September 2008. He had been referred there by his family physician for treatment of a bladder infection. However, he was left unattended in his wheelchair for more than 24 hours, and died 10 hours later, a subsequent inquest determining that "health-care workers from the hospital assumed Sinclair was drunk and 'sleeping it off' ... or was homeless and had come to avoid the cold". For some, however, that inquest did not go far enough. As one critic put it: "Medicine and health always sees itself as benevolent and caring for people. It's not true for many Indigenous people, it's a violent encounter," said Professor Barry Lavallee, in a CBC News report.[3] As others put it, Mr Sinclair was "ignored to death" because of racist attitudes towards an Indigenous person.[4]

What do we take from this sad story? One message is that Indigenous people in Canada have had, for years, poorer access to healthcare services than majority populations. Writers such as Dr Brenda Gunn claim that a "legacy of racial segregation in healthcare impacts the way Indigenous people encounter healthcare institutions as patients today".[5]

2. www.unicef.org/afghanistan/stories/female-health-workers-service-despite-countless-challenges
3. www.cbc.ca/news/canada/manitoba/winnipeg-brian-sinclair-report-1.4295996
4. www.ohchr.org/sites/default/files/Documents/Issues/IPeoples/EMRIP/Health/UniversityManitoba.pdf
5. Ibid., p. 4.

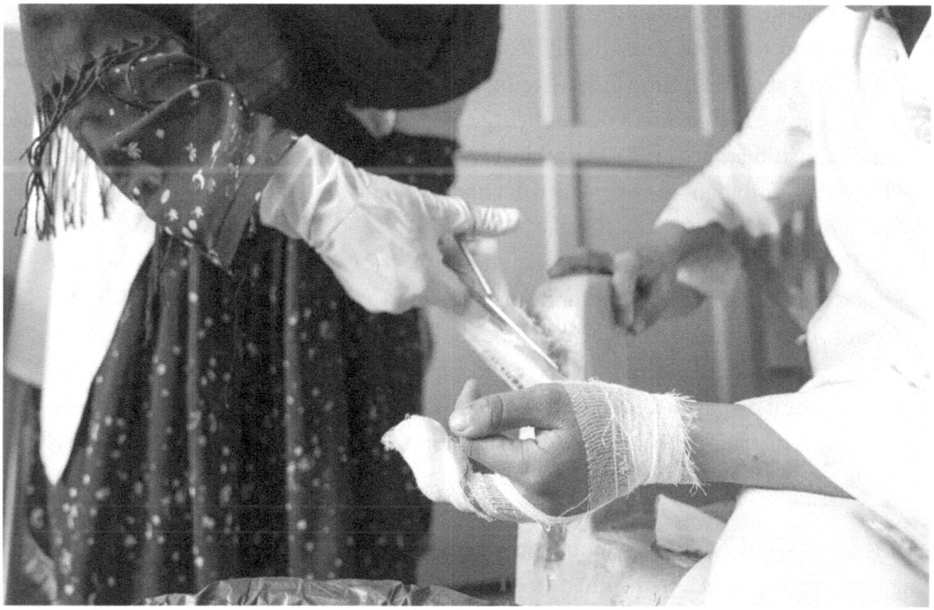

Figure 1.1 Nurse Sadia Khan dresses a wound
Source: UNICEF (2023).

We shall see later in this book other examples of racial discrimination, taken from the US, Australia and New Zealand. Another point is that hospitals are, ostensibly, places of care but such care may take unacceptably long to be delivered, whether because (as it appeared in Mr Sinclair's case) of discrimination or because resources (staffing, in particular) are inadequate to cope with demand. Regardless, Mr Sinclair was "care-less". Yet, lack of resources, and stigmatizing attitudes are not restricted to Indigenous peoples. Getting into a hospital is no guarantee of adequate care.

Here is a final story, extracted at some length from a wonderful book by the late doctor-anthropologist Paul Farmer (2020), relating to his work on the Ebola epidemic in Sierra Leone in 2014–15. The extract mentions four places in the country (Port Loko, Maforki, Hastings and the capital Freetown). Partners in Health[6] is the organization Farmer established to provide care in resource-poor countries.

> By the end of December, the size of the Partners in Health team in Port Loko [Figure 1.2] had grown close to eighty people, mostly nurses and doctors, but also logisticians and record keepers. Scores of sprayers and cleaners, most from around Port Loko and including several survivors, tried to keep the place clean

6. www.pih.org

> and supervised the donning and doffing of personal protective gear. A Cuban contingent of about forty finally reached Maforki. This meant that individual clinicians spent less time in sweltering protective gear. But even with their help, and what we hoped was a declining caseload, the Ebola victims who made long and punishing journeys to Maforki were sicker, and for longer, than those transferred by ambulances over short distances to Hastings from holding units in Freetown.
>
> Throughout the rest of the year, and into the next one, as the number of new cases at last began to fall, patients continued to reach Port Loko in terrible condition, often referred from far-off clinics or health posts and often having walked or been carried even to those. Ease and time of transportation explained some urban-rural disparities of outcome, but so did fear and confusion. Sick villagers had been instructed to avoid clinics and hospitals, but at the same time to report to them. (Farmer 2020: 127)

This piece speaks volumes about the geography of care, albeit in extremely challenging circumstances. As with other stories, it tells us that care involves an assemblage of elements, not only people – nurses, doctors, patients, ancillary workers – but non-human actors such as clinics, protective clothing, personal transport and ambulances, as

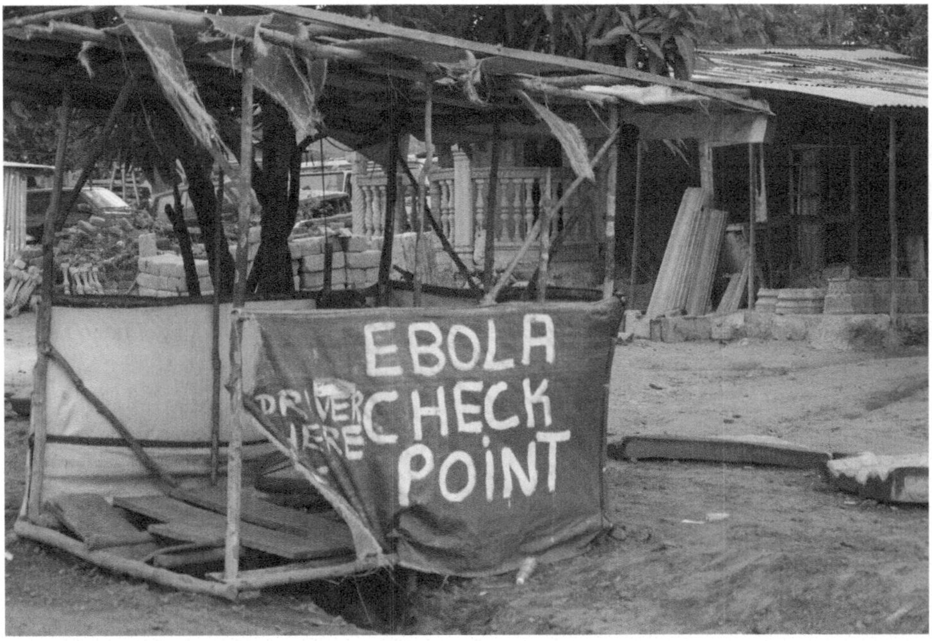

Figure 1.2 Port Loko, Sierra Leone, 2015
Source: iStock ID:478747934.

well as healthcare providers such as Partners in Health and those travelling from other countries (here, Cuba) to offer healthcare. All these elements have come together (been "assembled") to provide care for Ebola patients.

These four pieces are stories about very different people, situations and places. Despite differences in age, gender, ethnicity, material well-being and health status all these examples suggest that people require, or give, healthcare and that such care depends not only on their personal circumstances but on what is provided (or not) by the healthcare systems in the countries and regions where they live, as well as local provision and access to such provision. Further, while for Wendy her *utilization* of care takes place in a well-resourced country in the Global North, for nurse Sadia Khan in Afghanistan and those helping people suffering with Ebola, the *provision* of care is of a different order of magnitude in resource-poor countries in the Global South.

We are also reminded in all these stories that "care" is not merely a technical exercise (providing medicines, dressings and so on) but is infused with emotions too. Nurse Sadia clearly worries about her ability to provide *care*. Journeys are not merely the consumption of travel time but can be "punishing" (as for Ebola victims), while Wendy Davey was "terrified" about her wait for an ambulance. Whether providing or consuming care, people are neither automata dispensing it, nor human vessels waiting for something to be "done to" them. Feelings matter, and are shaped by both environments of care and the means of getting it delivered by and to people.

A further common feature of all four stories is mobility and, while this is a thread that runs throughout this book, it is given its own chapter. Wendy needed to get somewhere urgently. Sadia needs to get to work and her patients may not have the means to get to places for appropriate treatment. Brian was distinctly *im*mobile, left unattended in his wheelchair. Sierra Leoneans infected by Ebola moved, or were moved to, clinics that could offer care, while their carers too were mobile actors.

I want in this book to expand on the various issues raised by these four stories, all of which relate to varying degrees of unequal "access" (whether provision or utilization) to healthcare. Where possible, I shall focus on inequity and not simply inequality. The distinction matters. Inequalities in provision are differences or "disparities" (the word often used in the US literature). Inequities are differences that are potentially avoidable.

Having referred several times to "access" and (health)care, I need to unpack these and other concepts in the next chapter, which also considers the different approaches that geographers find it helpful to bring to bear on the subject.

2

GEOGRAPHIES OF ACCESS TO HEALTHCARE SERVICES

> We define access as the opportunity to identify healthcare needs, to seek healthcare services, to reach, to obtain or use health care services and to actually have the need for services fulfilled. Levesque *et al.* (2013: 8)

In this chapter I set out a range of approaches to describing and explaining access to healthcare services, from the perspective of a geographer. These modes of explanation, which are illustrated with various examples, might use either quantitative or qualitative methods, or perhaps a mix of the two. But before setting out these approaches I first consider the various places in which healthcare can be delivered and consumed. Some of these are formal settings (clinics, hospitals) but healthcare can of course be delivered elsewhere, not least in the home. This leads on to a wider discussion of the cultural dimension of such settings: landscapes of consumption, if you will. I then try to unpack what is meant by "access" to healthcare and show that there are various aspects of this, the main distinction being between *provision* of services and *utilization* of these services.

Places of healthcare

In this book I adopt a broad definition of healthcare services. A simple dictionary definition of the noun "service" is that it is the "action of helping or doing work for someone".[1] This does not say anything about who or what does the helping or work, nor does it suggest that the service might be provided for a group rather than an individual. My concern is with the systems, organizations and people who provide the "help" or "work" that maintains or improves people's health, and with those to whom such help or care is directed. I want to explore the geography of this healthcare and the extent to which it is delivered and accessed unequally across the globe, and within nation states and communities.

1. https://www.encyclopedia.com/social-sciences-and-law/law/law/service

Such giving of healthcare can involve many diverse settings, not only in the clinic or hospital. While a good deal of what follows in this book is concerned with treating illness or disease – how such treatments are provided and consumed in formal settings – healthcare can be, and is, delivered in other places. Power (2018) has an excellent introduction to the geography of care, and notes that care "is an enduring and contested concept in health *and* social support provision" (Power 2018: 96, my emphasis). The boundaries between "health" and "social" care are blurred. For example, emotional support, advice and assistance with shopping are all forms of support (or service, according to the dictionary) that are social but have impacts on the physical and mental health and well-being of others. Carers may be family members, close friends, volunteers, provided by charities or those employed by the state or private sector. I focus most of my attention on *healthcare* services and the systems within which they are embedded. To examine social care systems, social support and the full breadth of the geography of "care" requires a fuller treatment than is given here, although the final chapter does address the broader issue.

As suggested above, healthcare can take place in a variety of settings or places. Feeling unwell or "out of sorts" can be helped by rest or over-the-counter remedies, while those with a disability or chronic ill-health may be supported by family members or other carers, while remaining at home. But this is laden with inequality, perhaps due to income if wealthier people can afford more assistance, or by gender if the burden of help falls more on female family members (as is invariably the case: Seedat & Rondon 2021). Again, this is explored in the final chapter.

Formal healthcare provision is conventionally categorized as primary, secondary and tertiary. Primary healthcare includes both medical and non-medical services. The former includes visits to a general practitioner ("GP" in the UK, often "family physician" elsewhere) or nurse practitioner working in a clinic or health centre. Other settings provide dental healthcare or ophthalmic (eye) services, as well as community pharmacies. As the name suggests, primary care is a first "port of call". I shall have much to say later about unequal access to primary care, whether in rich countries (the Global North) or poorer countries (the Global South).

Secondary healthcare takes place in hospitals. The location and nature of these (whether large teaching hospitals or smaller facilities), relative to the populations they serve, inevitably calls for a geographical lens and this too is explored in later chapters. If such hospitals are highly specialized – for example, looking after people requiring transplants or other complex surgery – we speak of "tertiary" settings.

There are, however, other formal healthcare settings that do not fit neatly into this three-fold classification. For example, hospices are places providing palliative or end-of-life care; these too have fixed locations (although their services can be delivered to the home) and so there is a geography to such provision (see pp. 76–8). Another example would be so-called "traditional medicine" provided by and to many Indigenous groups and societies and which forms a key part of their cultures; this too is a form of primary healthcare. Some providers offer complementary and alternative forms of care (Brown *et al.* 2018: 83–4) that can be used alongside conventional medical healthcare.

Landscapes of (health)care and consumption

More broadly still, although not formal healthcare settings, there are many places that provide opportunities for well-being and recuperation and as such they have been explored by geographers. The best-known concept here is of the "therapeutic landscape", first introduced by Wil Gesler (1992) and the focus of edited books (e.g. Williams 2007) and dozens of examples. Therapeutic landscapes are places that provide for well-being, whether this be physical, emotional, spiritual or a combination of these. They might be quite ordinary settings, such as a private garden, nearby stream or public libraries (see Biglin 2021 for a compelling study of the engagement of refugees and asylum seekers with libraries in northern England). Gesler's original work explored iconic places such as the holy shrine at Lourdes in France, and spa towns such as Bath in England. Interestingly, and as pointed out by Gesler and Kearns (2002: 125–9), these places were "sold" or promoted through advertisements that painted a rosy picture of the potential health benefits that could be realized there. Treating care as a "commodity" – a theme discussed in several places in this book – is nothing new.

Led by early interventions from both Gesler and Robin Kearns (see, e.g., Gesler & Kearns 2002) geographers have for 25 years explored links between culture, place and health, but with a growing interest in care rather than formal healthcare settings. These authors have considered "consumption landscapes of care", including the "malling of medicine" in New Zealand and other countries, where walk-in clinics are "strategically located at consumer shopping hubs, and along major shopping streets and in shopping plazas" (Gesler & Kearns 2002: 144).

Further cultural, place-based research by these authors has explored the sorts of formal, clinical, healthcare settings that are the primary focus of this book. Gesler and Kearns (2002: 148) describe the Ascot Hospital in Auckland, New Zealand that opened in 1999; it is now part of a wider organization called MercyAscot Private Hospitals. Here, hospital rooms are "hotel spaces" and a current photograph (Figure 2.1) does indeed suggest that the hospital entrance looks more like a premier hotel. Ambience matters, quite aside from the high technology healthcare that is available to those that can afford it.

The Starship Hospital in Auckland, New Zealand, is a tertiary hospital centre dedicated to paediatric (children's) services. Opened in 1992, it aimed to "market the hospital as a distinctive place for monetary donors, as well as promoting a more potentially acceptable built environment for its youthful users" (Kearns & Barnett 2000: 84). Five years later the fast-food chain McDonald's opened a franchise on site, with hospital managers suggesting it normalized the hospital visit/stay for children while others lamented the

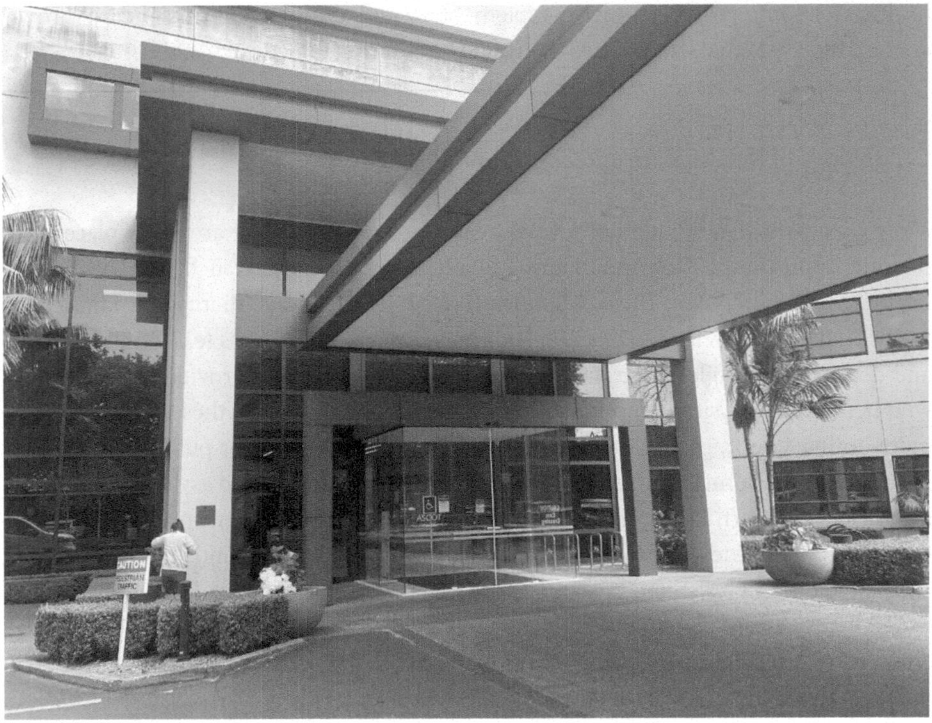

Figure 2.1 The entrance to the Ascot Hospital in Auckland, New Zealand
Source: Courtesy of Professor Robin Kearns, University of Auckland.

likelihood of increasing levels of obesity among children who love "happy meals". Kearns and Barnett (2000) see this co-location as symptomatic of the decline in the state funding of healthcare. They suggest that "arguments raised by adults concerning the unhealthy nature of McDonald's food essentially obscure deeper discourses surrounding the unpalatable character of the health reforms, particularly the commercialization of healthcare in New Zealand" (Kearns & Barnett 2000: 92). In 2005 McDonald's ceased operating at Starship. Celia Murphy, executive director of the Obesity Action Coalition, expressed her satisfaction: "Anything synonymous with chips and burgers is not appropriate in a health organisation anywhere, particularly a children's hospital".[2]

Some providers of hospital care prefer to engineer a clear spatial separation of the public and the commercial, with private provision "tucked away" within a larger hospital site. Indeed, some spaces within hospitals represent the very antithesis of commercialization and provide care that is very different from the medical interventions usually associated with those settings. Good examples are those places that provide social support, and sympathetic environmental and architectural design. To that end Martin

2. www.nzherald.co.nz/nz/mcdonalds-discharges-itself-after-eight-years-at-starship/3L57VLD2GR262CIC7HCEJ46FVY/

and Roe (2022) look at "Maggie's centres", cancer support settings in the UK that are located in regional oncology hospitals. The authors reveal how such spaces offer hope for people living with cancer, or their family members. As the authors put it, these centres "deliberately counteract the atmospherics of hospital environments, provide access to calming internal and outside spaces for their visitors, and use these in the delivery of their programme of care and support" (Martin & Roe 2022: 7). The same points can be made about hospices, and the provision and use of these is considered in Chapter 4.

Access to healthcare services

I have already referred to "access" but it is time to unpack the term. As we will see, it is a complex concept, which has exercised the attention of authors outside geography. In an important paper Ribot and Peluso (2003) defined access as the ability to derive benefit from things; such things including material objects, other people and institutions. They suggested it concerns "*who* does (and who does not) get to use *what*, in what ways, and *when*" (Ribot & Peluso 2003:154, my emphasis). To this list, as a geographer I would add "*where*".

Healthcare access has multiple meanings (Gulliford *et al.* 2002) and comprises several dimensions, but the key distinction is between *provision* and *utilization*. If there are sufficient services *provided* to meet healthcare needs then in principle people have access. Services have to be supplied in order for there to be any "access" at all; there has to be an "opportunity", whether it can be taken up or not. This is "potential" access (Aday & Andersen 1974; Gulliford *et al.* 2002: 186; Joseph & Phillips 1984: 58) and it is inherently geographical, since services have to be provided somewhere (usually in geographic space but sometimes on the move and often now virtually, in cyberspace). But the mere existence of a service is not sufficient; it has to be open or available when needed.

The second aspect is service *utilization* (or, simply, "use"), and this depends on the various barriers that are placed on those seeking services; such barriers may be organizational (the waiting times for consultation and/or treatment, for example), financial (costs of use, costs of travel, whether there is any insurance) or socio-cultural (the perceived acceptability of healthcare). Health service use is what Joseph and Phillips (1984: 2) call "revealed" access and Gulliford *et al.* (2002: 186) call "gaining access"; as they suggest, proof of access is use of services. This is also inherently geographical, since using healthcare services means "getting to them" (again, usually by overcoming geographic distance but sometimes in cyberspace using online consultations: see Chapter 7).

The relation between utilization and provision is sketched out in Figure 2.2, which reveals the structural determinants (both political/economic and spatial) and individual determinants of use, as well as the social context of health service consumption.

Similarly, Levesque *et al.* (2013) see access as the interface between potential service users and the characteristics of such service providers. As they put it: "access to healthcare is a product of supply factors, such as the location, availability, cost and appropriateness

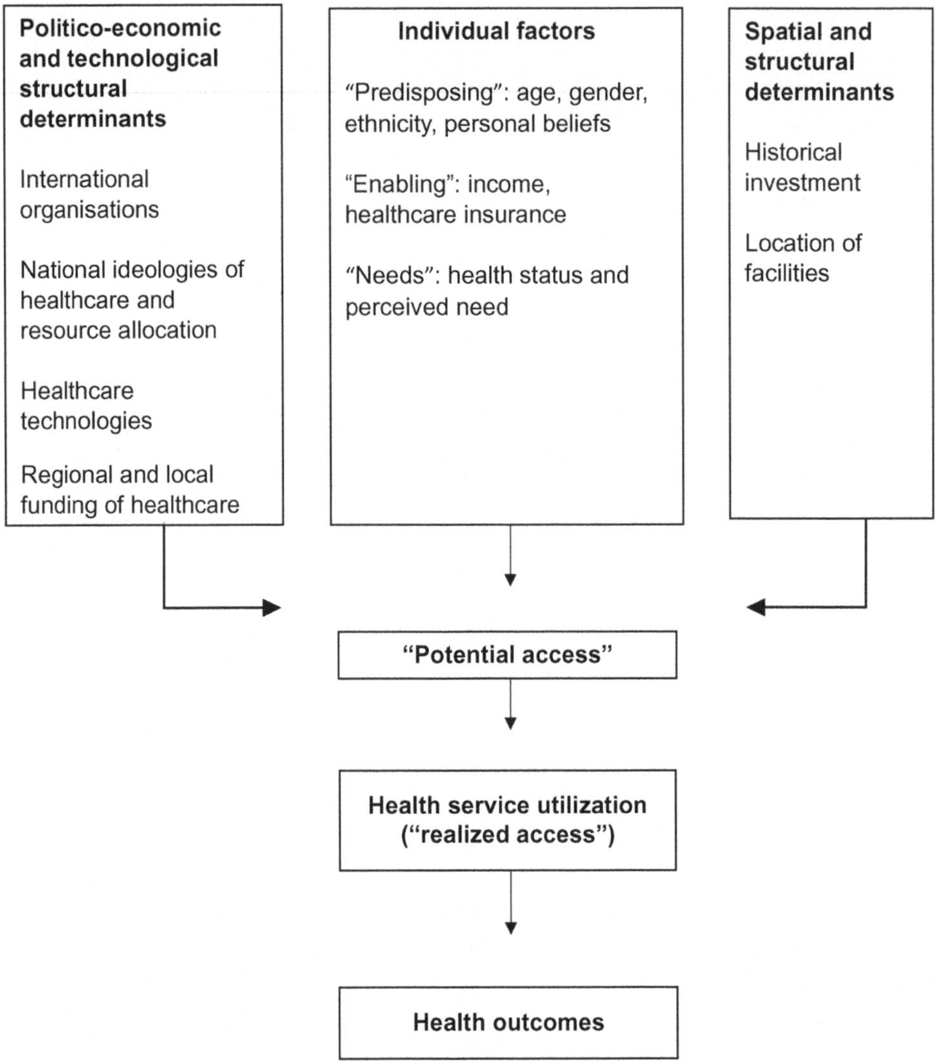

Figure 2.2 A model of healthcare access
Source: Based in part on Curtis (2004: 115) and Fiedler (1981: 130).

of services, as well as demand factors, such as the burden of disease and knowledge, attitudes and skills and self-care practices" (Levesque *et al.* 2013: 2). In simple terms, access is a function of both supply-side factors and demand for care.

Horrill and her colleagues (2018) consider many conceptualizations of access to be overly focused on the individual: their choices, their transport decisions, their education and so on. With a particular focus on Indigenous Canadians (see pp. 57–8) they prefer a postcolonial perspective, one that sees access less in terms of a service provision and more in terms of a social relationship. Here, "healthcare spaces are conceptualized as both clinical spaces and social spaces", the latter being the "invisible and contested space in which people from different social positions negotiate access to power and resources" (Horrill *et al.* 2018: 3). A postcolonial lens requires an examination of the historical, political and racial context within which healthcare provision has operated, and operates. Later chapters expand on some of these issues but, quite clearly, accessing healthcare is more than a function of individual behaviour (the predisposing, enabling and needs elements in Figure 2.2). Access depends upon structural properties of healthcare systems, including how and where these are provided, and on individual circumstances.

In an early paper Penchansky and Thomas (1981) identified five dimensions of access: *accessibility*, *availability*, *acceptability*, *affordability* and *adequacy* (also called *accommodation*) (see Brown *et al.* 2010: 521–39 and Saurman 2016 for more recent overviews). As Guagliardo (2004) has noted, the first two dimensions (accessibility and availability) are inherently geographical, since the former relates to the proximity of a service to a potential user and the latter relates to the resources to be found at the service. Consequently, Guagliardo brings the two together to speak of "spatial accessibility", and how this is measured is considered in the next section. Acceptability refers to consumer perception of the service, affordability to the direct costs incurred and adequacy to service organization (including, for example, waiting times). Saurman (2016) adds a sixth dimension: *awareness*, by which she means communication between provider and user.

For some authors access is also thought of in terms of outcomes. Gulliford and colleagues (2002: 187) say that "access could be measured using appropriate indicators of health status". However, this is rather unconventional and most authors would suggest that outcome (improved health or, worse, mortality) is *dependent on* access conceived in terms of provision and utilization. Gulliford *et al.* (2002: 188) also consider equity as an element of access. They write: "A concern to ensure that healthcare resources are mobilised to meet the needs of different groups in the population is *central to the concept of access*" (my emphasis). But equity is not itself a component of access; rather, a possible (and certainly desirable) result. As they themselves suggest, equity may, or may not, be assessed in terms of availability, utilization or outcomes.

Equity of access to healthcare is neatly summarized by the "inverse care law" (Box 2.1).

BOX 2.1 THE INVERSE CARE LAW

The inverse care "law", proposed by GP Julian Tudor Hart (1971; Figure 2.3), suggests that there is an inverse relationship between healthcare need and service provision. However, as a tribute to him when he died (in 2018, aged 91) John Lister wrote that:

> the concept can be read more broadly to argue that those with the greatest health needs are almost always those least able to afford the market price

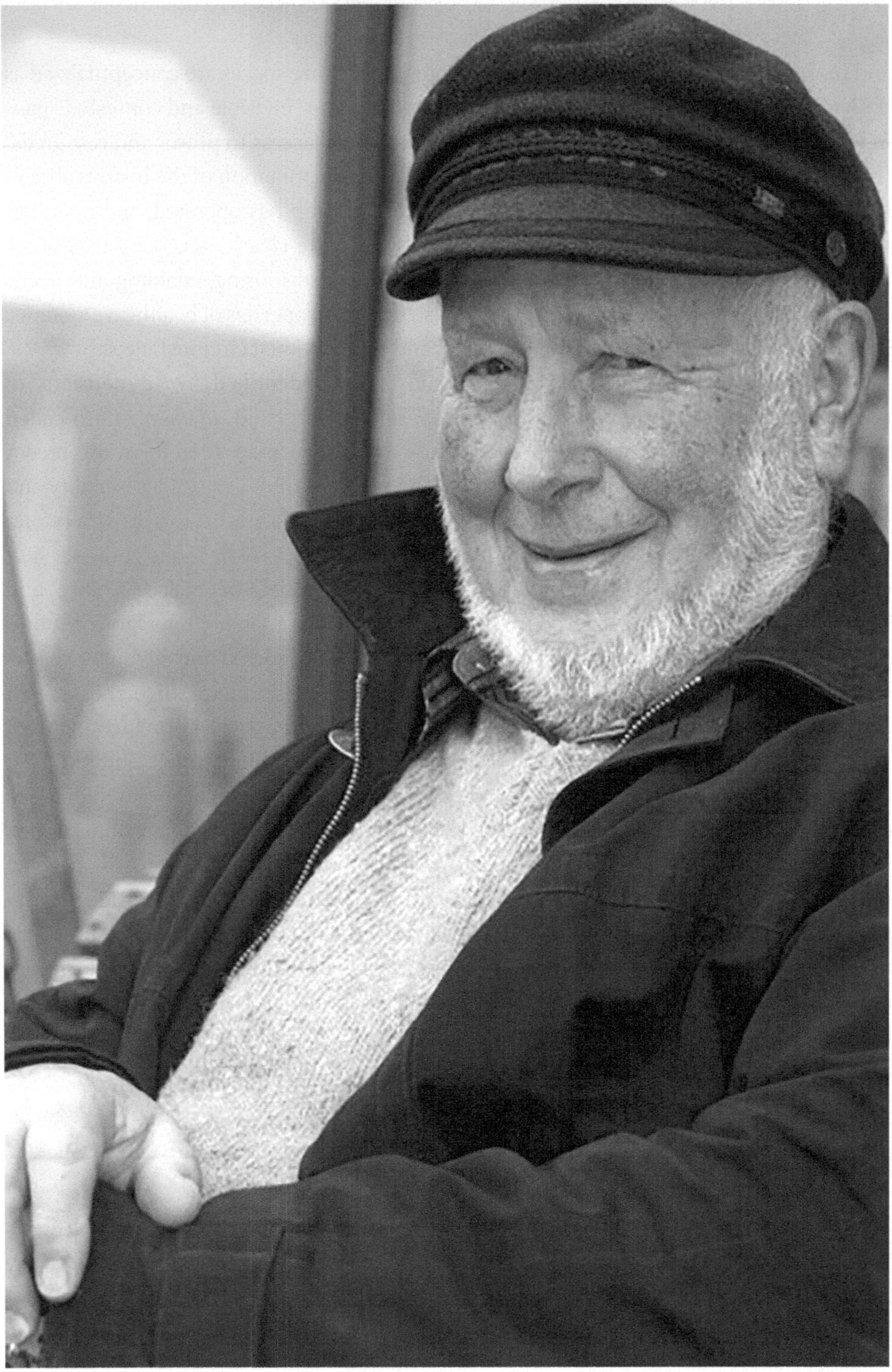

Figure 2.3 The late Dr Julian Tudor Hart
Source: Wikipedia.

of healthcare as a commodity; and it can explain why those areas facing the greatest deprivation are always those with the least political power to force change.[3]

Also writing in 2018, one of the most prolific writers on health inequity suggested that Tudor Hart's "seminal essay" remains as significant as it did when he wrote his landmark 1971 paper (Marmot 2018).

There is plenty of evidence from the UK and elsewhere that the geographical distribution of primary care clinics does not match the needs of patients, where "needs" are often measured by surrogate variables such as material deprivation. As Williams *et al.* (2004) observed, some practices in deprived areas have difficulties attracting doctors to work there. They also note that as well as the volume of staff working there we need a focus on the quality of provision. In England and Wales practices are eligible for "quality payments" if they meet certain standards. Williams's quantitative empirical work, conducted in South Wales, found that practices which offered training places for students and which were eligible for quality payments, were generally located in more affluent areas.

Examples of the inverse care law appear throughout this book, even if the "law" is not referred to explicitly.

I have said nothing about the "healthcare technologies" that form part of the structural determinants listed in Figure 2.2. I do so here with specific reference to the growing use of artificial intelligence (AI) in healthcare. Some of the issues are considered in Box 2.2 while further discussion of technologies is in Chapter 7.

Having unpacked what is meant by "access" to healthcare I turn to consider what approaches can be taken to explain the *geography* of such access. What distinctive contributions to our understanding of such access can geographers make?

Explaining geographies of access to healthcare

Gatrell and Elliott (2015) consider five contrasting approaches to the geography of health, and their usefulness in examining the geography of healthcare services more specifically is considered here. All five approaches have been used by researchers interested in provision and utilization, and while what follows is a brief summary – including an example of each – we shall see further examples in the chapters that follow. Different approaches focus attention on different components of the model presented in Figure 2.2, although some look at relations between them.

3. https://keepournhspublic.com/julian-tudor-hart-has-died-his-principles-live-on/

BOX 2.2 AI IN HEALTHCARE: ISSUES OF EQUITY

AI is "the ability of algorithms encoded in technology to learn from data so that they can perform automated tasks without every step in the process having to be programmed explicitly by a human" (WHO 2021: xi, cited in Shipton & Vitale 2024: 1). The same authors note that it is the latest in a series of technological innovations in healthcare; like all such innovations it necessitates a critical examination.

Some authors are guilty of exaggerating its role. Garcia-Saiso *et al.* (2024: 2) note that "AI can analyze health service utilization patterns to identify inequalities in access to care". Yet, as we see below, we do not need AI to do this; the geographical tools to identify such inequalities have long been available and we shall see several examples in this book. These authors also conflate AI with existing digital technologies. "AI-powered applications can remind patients about medication schedules, appointments, and health check-ups, especially helping those with limited access to regular health care". They go on to suggest that "AI can optimize resource allocation, route planning for ambulances". But operations research tools to do this have been used for over 60 years by geographers (see, e.g., Cromley & McLafferty 2011). As we see in Chapter 7 these technologies have been in place well before AI became fashionable; there has to be more to AI than the use of information technology!

Those authors who have adopted a more critical appraisal note that AI requires large data sets for "training"; but if these data privilege one group over another the outputs will be biased (Nordling 2019). Simply put, if the training data come from research on white male populations it will lead to predictions that are hardly likely to be applicable to non-white female groups. There is therefore possible contextual bias such that (for example) the algorithms devised for those living in the Global North may not be generalizable to those living in the Global South.

Having said that, AI can be of value in resource-poor – and rural – areas where there may be a lack of expert clinicians available to identify people with specific conditions and diseases. However, even in these areas there needs to be the infrastructure (at the most basic level, good electricity and internet connectivity) in place to read and interpret any evidence supplied by AI tools.

The most critical examination of AI in healthcare comes from those who argue that "technological interventions without political change reinforce the multiple intersections of power that structure health care, such as racism, patriarchy, and neoliberalism" (Shipton & Vitale 2024: 2). Those actors who collect and have access to large data sets can exercise considerable power. Further, framing AI as a solution to workforce shortages ignores the political economy of a lack of healthcare professionals, particularly in the Global South. We consider such shortages below (pp. 63–7).

Writing in 2026 such a critical account may turn out to be misplaced. Time will tell.

Positivist approaches

Very simply put, to describe a geographic study as "positivist" means that it is concerned with spatial arrangement, and uses quantitative methods (mathematics and statistics) to describe and model such patterns (Cresswell 2024: 80–85). In a healthcare context it means looking at the location of healthcare facilities and the spatial distribution of potential service users, then mapping and measuring the relative location of such users and the facilities. There are dozens of empirical studies exploring whether increased distance from healthcare facilities results in their being less used, other factors being equal (the classic text is Joseph & Phillips 1984). Most such studies look at a regional or local context, but some authors have produced high-resolution regional and global maps of travel time to healthcare facilities (Box 2.3). Geldsetzer and colleagues (2020) have done so for countries in sub-Saharan Africa, with particular reference to access for older adults. Wigley and colleagues (2020) have measured the availability and geographical accessibility of maternity services, also across sub-Saharan Africa.

BOX 2.3 MAPPING TRAVEL TIME TO HEALTHCARE FACILITIES AT THE GLOBAL SCALE

Weiss *et al.* (2020) have constructed a global dataset of the locations of healthcare facilities (hospitals and clinics) using data from Google Maps and OpenStreetMap. This reveals the number of such facilities (both public and private) in over 376,000 1 km square pixels (most of which, of course, have no such facility since many grid squares are in isolated rural areas). Data on roads and road speed data were combined with these locations and shortest-distance algorithms used to estimate journey times (using both motorized transport but also walking) from each pixel to the nearest facility. Such travel time maps are overlaid with gridded population data to provide estimates of the percentage of the world's population within one hour of a facility – either by vehicle or on foot. Results show that about 60 per cent of the world's population live within 10 minutes of a hospital or clinic if they have access to motorized transport, and over 90 per cent live within an hour's drive. In contrast, for those walking only 57 per cent live within an hour from a facility. As the authors acknowledge, simply being within a travel time window does not guarantee that the facility is open or affordable, nor do the data reveal anything about the nature and range of provision.

Some authors have developed this further to examine not simply potential access but revealed or actual service usage. Gligorić and her colleagues (2023) use anonymized smartphone location history data for over 100 countries and find that the potential access revealed by Weiss and colleagues, and other studies, underestimate considerably the actual travel times incurred by service users. For half the countries studied the differences between revealed and potential travel times is over 60 minutes. There are of course considerable within-country variations. For example, in Nigeria the average travel time to a facility by motor vehicle is 41 minutes, but 10 per cent of users travel more than three hours to access care.

These studies have, to an extent, advanced our knowledge of spatial accessibility at a global scale. Inevitably, however, these very broad-brush approaches cannot help us understand the experiences of service users or the other dimensions of access portrayed in Figure 2.2.

Planning the locations of healthcare facilities is clearly a matter of geography, since such facilities have to be located *somewhere* (I defer to Chapter 7 the issue of provision "on the move" and so-called "telehealthcare"). For over 60 years geographers have worked on models for the optimal spatial allocation of healthcare facilities (see Abler *et al.* 1971 for a clear introduction to some classic methods, and Brown *et al.* 2010: 540–66 and Cromley & McLafferty 2011, for more recent summaries). The question however is, "optimal" for whom? From the perspective of potential service users, it is desirable to have a relatively large number of facilities (such as primary care centres or hospitals) within easy reach. That might also be attractive to those working there, whether clinicians or other staff, who will prefer shorter journeys to work. Yet from the perspective of governments, national and regional, who have to fund these facilities, it might be preferable to have a smaller set of such facilities that allow for economies of scale and scope. Potential service users might also find it more optimal to visit large centres that have "state of the art" facilities and accompanying expertise, knowing that (in principle at least) they may get better care there than in a more local setting. There are, then, relative advantages and disadvantages of concentration and dispersal of healthcare (Gatrell & Elliott 2015: 193–4). This issue is considered further in Chapter 3, with regard to cancer services.

As noted above, a distinctive geographic contribution to understanding access to healthcare services is to measure spatial accessibility. This requires information on: the population(s) requiring a service; characteristics of service supply; and spatial separation of consumers from services. The latter can be measured using straight-line distances or, more usefully, road distances or travel times (as in Box 2.3). Service supply depends on whether we are looking at primary or hospital-based care, but could be represented by data on the number of clinicians employed at a particular facility. Population demand depends on the particular context and might be total population, or a subset thereof.

The most common method of bringing these three components together is known as the "two-step floating catchment area" solution (2SFCA; Box 2.4).

BOX 2.4 MEASURING SPATIAL ACCESSIBILITY USING THE "TWO-STEP FLOATING CATCHMENT AREA" (2SFCA) MODEL

A first step in the 2SFCA method is to compute the ratio of supply to demand at a particular health centre. "Supply" might be taken to be the number of healthcare professionals working in a centre. "Demand" for care may be measured by the population residing within a fixed distance or travel time to that centre (the catchment area). The second step is, for each residential area (such as a census tract), to identify all facilities within the threshold distance (drive time) and to sum their supply–demand ratios. This yields a spatial accessibility score for that area; such scores can be mapped to give a cartographic representation of healthcare accessibility.

This approach was first adopted in a healthcare context by Luo and Wang (2003) but it has also been modified in a number of ways. For example, rather than simply adding up the populations living with a fixed distance of a facility, some weighting of population can be applied to acknowledge "distance decay effects" (where those living closer to a centre may have greater "demand").

The 2SFCA method (and subsequent modifications) has been widely adopted. For example, Chen *et al.* (2023) analysed the spatial accessibility to healthcare centres in the city of Shenzhen, part of Guangdong province in south-eastern China. The supply side was measured by the number of healthcare "technicians" (including doctors, nurses and pharmacists) per head of population. Demand was simply the census population in each of 771 communities, while spatial separation was measured by road travel time. As an aside, Chen *et al.* (2023) also determine a set of optimal locations for healthcare facilities in Shenzhen. The authors suggest that their work helps to support the promotion of equitable access to primary healthcare services in the Shenzhen city region. In related work in the same region, Tao *et al.* (2020) classified the facilities into primary, secondary and tertiary centres (612, 35 and 19 respectively). The number of physicians working in each represented "supply" and a modified version of the 2SFCA method was used to incorporate the hierarchical nature of healthcare provision. Results (Figure 2.4) suggest considerable unevenness in provision.

For further updates of floating catchment area models see Kim *et al.* (2018) and, more recently, Jörg and Haldimann (2023). Yu and colleagues (2024) suggest that modelled travel times often underestimate actual travel times (assessed using smartphone data) to healthcare facilities.

A widely used method in health geography is multilevel modelling which, put simply, explains health outcomes in terms of "compositional" factors (the nature of places) and "contextual" factors (the characteristics of people living in such places) (see Gatrell & Elliott 2015: 78–86, for a brief outline). The method has also been used to model the utilization of healthcare. A good example is research by Mulyanto *et al.* (2019) in Indonesia.

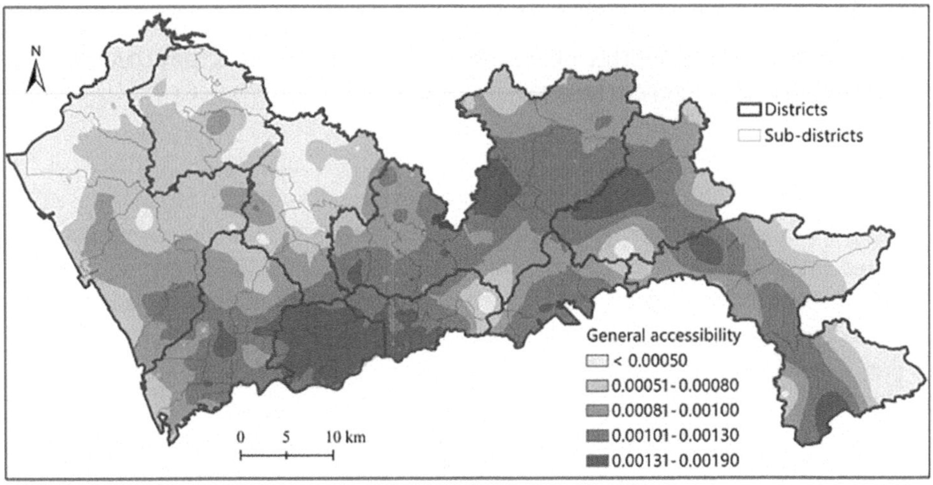

Figure 2.4 Accessibility of healthcare facilities in Shenzhen, China
Source: Tao *et al.* (2020).

Hospital use by almost 650,000 adults was related to the areas (districts and provinces) in which they lived, where "context" was measured by level of urbanization and population density. "Compositional" factors included wealth, education and insurance status. Results suggested that "context" was more important than "composition". Districts in the Java region had higher hospital use than those in other regions, and utilization was higher in city districts. Service availability explained more of the variation in hospital utilization than did individual factors such as insurance.

Multilevel modelling has also been used to study geographic inequalities in access to transgender healthcare (Box 2.5).

These sorts of "positivist" studies have value in the sense that they can identify areas of relatively poor service provision as well as which communities are underserved, as illustrated in a study set in a small region of Tanzania (Kimario *et al.* 2024). Such research can potentially aid planners in making decisions about additional investment, although such decisions are more likely to be made with a political mindset rather than with community interest. What positivist studies lack, therefore, is an understanding of the political context and the perspectives of those people and communities who are potential users of healthcare facilities.

Social interactionist approaches

In acknowledgement of the importance of the human and community voice we can consider approaches – here termed "social interactionist" – that reveal some of the factors that explain potential access and the experience of using healthcare facilities.

BOX 2.5 TRANSGENDER HEALTHCARE

Transgender people have a gender identity that differs from the sex they were assigned at birth. Poor access to appropriate healthcare for transgender people is linked to worse mental health as well as suicidal thoughts, particularly among young people. Such access is geographically uneven, particularly in the US, where 26 states have policies, or have passed legislation, restricting access. Those states that do not have policies protecting transgender people tend to have a higher percentage of people voting Republican (Hughto *et al.* 2016). Borah *et al.* (2023) have estimated that 89,000 transgender youths (aged 13–17 years) live in states that have restricted gender-affirming medical care. Drive times to gender clinics before restrictions were placed on access averaged about half an hour, but this rose to almost one hour after restrictions were enacted.

Using national survey data for almost 6,000 transgender adults Hughto *et al.* (2016) modelled clinical refusal of care as a function of both individual and geographic factors. Their multilevel model found that older people, those on low incomes and people of colour were more likely to be refused care. Geographically, people living in southern and western states were more likely to be denied care; specifically, these states were: Florida, Arizona, Tennessee, Oregon, Arkansas, Alaska, Connecticut, North Dakota, Oklahoma and Idaho. Everhart and colleagues (2023) use a modified version of the floating catchment area method to examine access to transgender hormone therapy in Texas. Their results identify areas, such as parts of Fort Worth and Dallas, where transgender care provision is poor.

These kinds of analysis tell us nothing about the emotional costs of denying access to such care. We need other approaches, such as those discussed in the following sections, to illuminate the human dimension. For an important study that traces the pathway from primary care to specialist gender identity clinics in England and Wales see Wright *et al.* (2021).

Gatrell and Elliott (2015: 37–41) give more details, and examples, of what is meant by this approach but in essence it is concerned with the meanings that people give to their health or their interactions (conversations or encounters) with healthcare providers. In the chapters that follow we will see several examples of this kind of research, but for now we consider research that follows neatly from the quantitative "distance-based" studies considered previously.

Much research points to the relative absence of healthcare providers (especially obstetricians and gynaecologists) in rural areas, which have been characterized as "healthcare deserts" (we return in Chapter 4 to the issues of medically underserved areas). Statz and Evers (2020) undertook a study in rural Minnesota that included interviews with 51 women: both service providers and potential service users. In a telling extract the authors argue that "truly no one understands rural distance better than those who have to traverse it ... no-one is more qualified to evaluate distance amid the full extent of rural healthcare deserts than rural women" (Statz & Evers 2020: 3). Barriers to accessing healthcare among this group were not merely spatial but included some of the issues depicted in Figure 2.2, notably lack of insurance but also whether there was access to a car (and the means to fill it up for a long return journey). The stress involved meant that some women decided not to access care. Those able to visit relatively close facilities expressed frustration that they did not see a qualified physician/doctor but instead a less well-qualified associate. Some women travel considerable distances to see a doctor they trust, subverting the usual finding that utilization decreases with increasing distance. The authors conclude: "In conjunction with the sociospatial barriers rural women report, the interpersonal costs of physician shortages, insufficient payment models, and an increasingly stressed and limited health system create negative experiences that compound rural women's ability and willingness to seek care" (Statz & Evers 2020: 5).

Interviews with 25 people (mostly women) living in rural Missouri (Kukulka *et al.* 2024) suggested attitudes of self-sufficiency for care, along with negative views of local healthcare providers. For example, one participant said: "*If you need something done ... you have to leave [rural area] to get it done properly. People usually say, if you stop at our hospital, your next step is going to a funeral home*". Another said: "*If you ever [get bucked off a horse], [you] get back on ... You're not a sissy on a farm*". But the authors conclude that although their study "underscores the importance of cultural values and promoting patient directed care, structural barriers remain at the forefront of discussions about healthcare utilization in rural communities" (Kulkuka *et al.* 2024: 5). These remarks, and the work of Statz and Evers, suggest that we need to consider more than human "agency". There are structural determinants of access to healthcare, as we see in the next section.

Kwiringira and colleagues (2021) undertook a study of health service access on the Kalangala islands of Lake Victoria, Uganda. Although they are interested in geographical accessibility they explore the intersections of this with social factors, drawing on interviews with service users and district health officers. Since there are 84 islands, most having no health facility, there are challenges in meeting healthcare needs, people requiring lengthy journeys from island to island (or mainland). As one islander put it:

> *Even if you have all the money in the world, once the lake is turbulent, you cannot travel ... here we only go for treatment when we have money because it is a season for fish and therefore, we have money, but also when the lake is calm. We have lost some people because the lake was not navigable.*
>
> (in Kwiringira *et al.* 2021: 4)

However, such geographical challenges (the "contextual" factors mentioned earlier) are compounded by the social ("compositional") challenges faced by islanders and workers. The authors describe a "risk culture", particularly among fishermen, where informal sexual relations are normalized and testing for HIV is patchy.

In Bengaluru (formerly Bangalore), India, Patil and colleagues (2023) explore the transport inequalities faced by older adults who need to access healthcare. Sixty interviews were conducted, all during the Covid-19 pandemic. As with the previous study, personal circumstances intersect with transport systems, whether by bus, car or on foot (or a combination of these). Those living on the periphery of this major city (the third largest in India) were at a particular disadvantage given that most hospitals were in or near the city centre. Some users needed multiple modes of transport. As one 62-year-old man said: "*I have to take an auto and go to Nayandahalli metro station and from there I take the metro and again I will take an auto to reach the hospital*" (Patil *et al.* 2023: 7). The journey is made even harder by the lack of consideration given by other transport users. A 70-year-old woman explains: "*I get in and stand all the while. There is seating arrangement for senior citizens, but they do not give place … When I am tired it is usually very difficult to stand. What to do? Conductors can help but they won't*" (ibid.: 7). These "mobility" challenges are discussed further in Chapter 7.

There are many stories to be told about, and by, transgender people. British psychology student Nikki Hayden says wistfully: "*Trans people are the same as everyone else, our ideals in life are to be happy, to be respected, to be comfortable*".[4] These ideals contrast with widespread experience of stigma and poor access to healthcare, some of which depends on where trans people live. An illustration of this comes from New Zealand, where:

> the inconsistencies across New Zealand's 20 district health boards (DHBs) are stark. In one area, a person's GP may be able to prescribe hormones, but if that same person was to live elsewhere, they might have to wait months to visit an endocrinologist who specialises in hormone treatment first.[5]

Growing up in a very rural part of the South Island, "Krystal" had a GP who knew nothing about trans healthcare but did eventually refer her to an endocrinologist in Dunedin, a four-hour return trip from her home. Krystal tells us: "*My life's been incredibly hell. I don't know how I managed to live like this, but I have. I'm so, so lonely*". She feels she must relocate: "*I'm actually moving to Christchurch in April and I have to give up everything that I've got down here just for this transition, because there's no help down here*".

4. www.theguardian.com/society/2016/jul/10/transgender-stories-people-think-we-wake-up-and-decide-to-be-trans
5. www.rnz.co.nz/programmes/here-we-are/story/2018773670/trans-healthcare-a-harmful-postcode-lottery

Elsewhere on the South Island, Leo tells us: "*It makes me feel like being trans is some medical fault that needs fixing. It makes me feel like my understanding of my own gender isn't enough*".

Only the most heartless could fail to be moved by these stories.

Structuralist approaches

As is clear from Figure 2.2 there are "politico-economic and technological structural determinants" of healthcare access. To shed light on these, and to go beyond individualistic or behavioural approaches, we need to draw on political economy or "structuralist" perspectives. The latter can include both Marxist and critical feminist explanations, since both embrace conflict or power relations, whether between social classes or gender. Power is distributed unequally, with a capitalist class exercising domination over a working class, or with men exercising domination over women.

A political economy perspective concerns itself with production, distribution and consumption. In a healthcare context this means examining how services are produced by the state, how resources are allocated (for example, devolved to regional or local organizations) and how they are made available to consumers. More commonly, a political economy perspective has been used to explain health inequalities; however, my concern here is with how it can inform our understanding of the provision and use of healthcare. This will be examined in more detail in Chapter 3, where we consider the different roles played by the state (and international organizations) as opposed to market forces.

Key to an understanding of contemporary political economy is neoliberalism, promoted by Chicago economists led by Milton Friedman, pursued by the World Bank and the International Monetary Fund (IMF), and implemented in the US by President Reagan and in the UK by Margaret Thatcher (Boyle 2021: 106–12). The consequences for healthcare, across the globe, have been profound, since the effect of neoliberalist policies, such as structural adjustment programmes ("SAPs": see Gatrell 2023: 77–8), has been to replace public welfare with private markets and reduced taxation that have served to increase inequality and austerity.

Among many examples, Sakellariou and Rotarou (2017) consider the impact of neoliberalism on access to healthcare for people with disabilities in both Chile and Greece. Under the dictator General (and former geographer) Augusto Pinochet, who had displaced President (and former doctor) Salvador Allende in 1973, the healthcare system was substantially restructured, with cuts to public health budgets and the promotion of private health insurance. In Greece, the impact of the global financial crisis in 2007–08 was to have imposed the conditions of structural adjustment or "bailout" by the IMF and a reduction in healthcare expenditure, including that on cancer services and mental health. For people with disabilities, often on low incomes or without employment, such neoliberal policies have particularly significant impacts. Sakellariou and Rotarou (2017) consider such effects as a form of "structural violence" (see Gatrell 2023: 2–3): the destructive impact inflicted by those exercising power or domination over a weaker group.

Porter (2013) analysed the impact, both in the UK and US, of austerity measures that followed the same financial crisis (2007–08). As has been pointed out by others (e.g. Stuckler *et al.* 2017) the burden of these measures – reductions in public spending – fell on the poor. More concretely, in the UK NHS hospitals were required to make "efficiency savings". In the US, attempts by the Obama administration (2009–17) to restructure healthcare along a more "socialized" European model was resisted by the interests of financial capital in the form of healthcare insurance companies. Porter points out that "neoliberalism has definitively replaced welfarism as the dominant ideology" (Porter 2013: 13). He continues (14): "Healthcare systems, especially those that had been socialized during the period of welfare economics, have become rich pickings for the ever-more confident bourgeoisie". These assertions are examined more fully in the following chapter.

What of feminist perspectives on access to healthcare that can also be labelled "structuralist" because of their emphasis on power relations? A "materialist" feminism stresses how bureaucracy, policies, regulations and so on constrain access to healthcare for women. A "critical" feminism adds a concern with how other dimensions of identity, including race, class, disability and sexuality, "intersect" with gender (see Cresswell 2024: 164–6 on "intersectionality"). Such biased healthcare access may well be implicit rather than overt, but it is nonetheless real. A feminist argument is that poor health outcomes for women arise from patriarchal structures within capitalist society, which constrain women's equal access to the resources they need.

To make this more concrete we can point to large-scale restructuring of healthcare systems that have taken some care out of the hospital setting and into the home. Hospital managers are invariably keen to discharge patients into the "community" but what that means is shifting care into the private space of the home and, usually, having women undertake the (unpaid) labour of care. A good example of this comes from a study undertaken by Brassolotto and Daly (2016). These authors adopt the framework of feminist political economy to explore the care given in the home to people on dialysis (for renal disease). Such demanding work has implications for those doing the caring, including sacrificing their own hobbies and neglecting their own health. The authors' specific focus is rural British Columbia, where centralization of services has placed more of the care burden on the domestic environment and in particular, women. While some training on home dialysis is available, this hardly compensates for the lengthy training that health professionals receive. Further, those on very low incomes could not afford respite care, paid companions or assistance from the private sector. The authors' feminist political economy lens illustrates that "a consequence of shifting treatment from the clinic to the home is the substantial amount of invisible work, costs, and responsibility transferred from institutions to patients and their families" (Brassolotto & Daly 2016: 528). We consider these issues further in Chapter 8.

Structurationist approaches

Curtis (2004: 116) argues that "individual level factors interact with structural aspects of the local social milieu, the local health service organization and policy and the spatial structures of local facilities for the delivery of healthcare". In other words, human agency works alongside structures of healthcare systems to explain access (see Figure 2.2). Further, as we see in Chapter 3, the "local" to which Curtis refers is also, to varying degrees, shaped by national and international policies.

The interaction between structure and agency demands an approach that considers both together and this approach can be labelled "structurationist" (Gatrell & Elliott 2015: 50–53; Cresswell 2024: 194–201), a term coined by British sociologist Anthony Giddens. Giddens drew upon time-geography, formulated by the Swedish geographer Torsten Hägerstrand (Cresswell 2024: 195–6: see also Gatrell & Elliott 2015: 51), which maps how people move through space during a particular time period (a day, maybe a year). While people may be able to exercise choice (agency) in how and where they move, they are *constrained* by "structures" of various kinds. In a healthcare context such constraints could be the relative locations of facilities and thus the distances they have to travel, as well as the opening times of clinics. To give a simple example, you might want treatment for a worrying skin infection and seek an appointment with a GP (in a British context) or general physician. But if an appointment is unavailable you might head to an Accident and Emergency (A&E) department at a hospital (an Emergency Room: ER), knowing it is open 24 hours a day. Whether this is a good use of A&E is matter of opinion but people may make that choice if they perceive constraints on the availability of care elsewhere.

Some of the spatial accessibility studies referred to earlier imply that people may have potential access to more than one healthcare facility and can exercise choice. But choice is invariably limited. In the UK, for example, a general practice can refuse patients if there are "reasonable grounds" (for example if you live outside the area that the surgery covers). In other words, "choice" is constrained by relative location – where you live. Further, while in the UK, and many other countries, you can "choose" whether to use services provided by the state, or those offered by private providers, this is hardly much of a choice for those on low incomes.

As Cresswell (2024: 198) notes, structuration has much in common with the work of the French sociologist Pierre Bourdieu. Among many of his key concepts are those of the "field" and different forms of "capital". We can conceive of healthcare as a "field" of activity, as suggested by Collyer *et al.* (2017: 98). They argue as follows:

> Given that, by definition, all fields are sites of struggle, and are constituted by a set of relations between a range of positions that reproduce the field itself analysis should proceed by identifying the key actors and the relations between the positions in which these actors stand.

In the healthcare field such actors include health professionals, health organizations, insurance providers and researchers, although some geographers would broaden this out to include technologies, materials and other entities that form the "assemblages" referred to in Chapter 1. Collyer (2017: 99) argues that the healthcare field "is fundamentally capitalist, for [it] is provided amidst a complexity of relations between the private and public sectors, and an on-going tension between the treatment of health and healthcare as a commodity versus a right of citizenship".

Following Bourdieu further, the individual factors identified in Figure 2.2 can be conceptualized in terms of the nature and volume of different forms of "capital", as follows:

- economic capital: travel costs, or to pay for treatment or insurance;
- social capital: support networks and social influences;
- cultural capital: level and type of education, including health beliefs and preferences.

Paccoud *et al.* (2020) have explored these different forms of capital in a healthcare context, with reference to older adults. Different forms of capital are potentially exchangeable with each other: economic capital can be used to enable mobility, and social capital can for example help accumulate cultural capital if friends can help inform people about healthcare opportunities, thereby easing their access to healthcare. People with lower stocks of different forms of capital may use healthcare less than those with higher stocks who may be more strategic in its use, perhaps seeking to prevent ill-health before the need for intervention arises.

In their empirical work (across several European countries, involving 65,000 older adults) Paccoud *et al.* (2020) operationalize these different forms of capital. For example, economic capital is measured using total household wealth; cultural capital uses data on level of education; and social capital is represented by level of participation in social activities (such as clubs and societies). Using statistical methods, they show that economic capital has the largest effect on contact with a health professional or with a dentist but all three types play a significant role. Such a quantitative study puts some flesh on the bones of the conceptual model presented in Figure 2.2.

To Bourdieu's different forms of capital, we could add "health" or "physical" capital – one's own health status – since this too is a determinant of use. Further, we can speak of "mobility capital" (sometimes called "motility"), which Kaufmann *et al.* (2004: 750) suggest refers to how people "access and appropriate the capacity for socio-spatial mobility according to their circumstances"; see Chapter 7). In doing so we see a link back to notions of time-geography and the different abilities people have to traverse space in order to access healthcare.

All these different forms of capital are unequally distributed among individuals and social groups.

Post-structuralist approaches

Post-structuralism is a set of perspectives that (as the prefix "post" suggests) does away with suppositions that macro-level forces or structures determine social life. It is, as Cresswell (2024: 209) puts it, "happy to stay at the surface of life rather than digging for deeper 'truth'". As far as geographers are concerned, it means looking at space not as a container of objects (such as the location of healthcare facilities) but as a set of relations between diverse objects that coalesce into networks of various kinds. This is far removed from simply looking at access in terms of distance from place of residence to place of care.

In an important paper that illustrates one post-structuralist approach, Stoller (2003) explores how women are able (or not) to access healthcare in prison. "In prison healthcare, the correctional system and its punitive discourse combine to increase the social, psychological, and emotional distance between the care provider and the recipient" (Stoller 2003: 2274). Drawing on the stories of individual prisoners, Stoller shows how incarcerated women seek care that may be provided by sympathetic caregivers, but both prisoner and health worker are "institutionally thwarted in their attempts to reach each other". The prisoner's mobility, and therefore access to healthcare, is inevitably constrained and controlled by prison rules and discipline. As Stoller puts it: "where humanistic health practice requires an acknowledgment of interconnectedness, prisons are based on principles of exclusion, separation, and confinement" (Stoller 2003: 2265). Even within the confines of a prison, the particular prisoner about whom she speaks draws on a social network of fellow inmates who do their best to help her access healthcare. The difficulties of getting an appointment to see a health professional apply as much to the prisoner as to someone not imprisoned, but there is little or no choice in who she gets to consult with. We can see that the determinants of access to healthcare (Figure 2.2) are writ large for prisoners.

Stoller also speaks of the "objects in prison space: in addition to the beds, the keys, the doors, and ducats (movement passes) of prison life, there are the wheelchair, the equipment for emergencies, and the pill envelopes of the medical system" (Stoller 2003: 2270). This brings to mind another type of post-structuralist account, that dealing with the assemblages referred to above: the fact that these different elements (or "actors") come together to form a "network" that impacts on how healthcare is accessed. In an interesting exploration of assemblages, Cresswell (2024: 217) uses the example of street markets which "exuberantly bring things (food, clothes, smells, sounds) together alongside stories and symbols and the practices of buying, selling, and performing". Much the same could be said of a private hospital or clinic, albeit with the need to add the technical components. If we do so we can start to speak of an "actor-network".

Some researchers have drawn on actor network theory (ANT) to describe service provision. For example, Usher and Denis (2022) examined how, in an urban neighbourhood in Québec, different interest groups (minorities, older adults, immigrants) came together to influence healthcare provision. However, the network elements were people and it would appear that the analysis is more of a "social network" approach rather than one drawing on the non-human (mostly technical) actors that a more conventional ANT approach would suggest. Although not concerned with health service provision, an interesting paper by Yan and He (2020) uses ANT to explore links between health tourism and the therapeutic landscapes referred to earlier (p. 9).

Stoller (2003) drew on the work of Michel Foucault, whose own work on prisons as disciplinary spaces has become well-known to geographers. Key concepts in Foucault's work are "governmentality" and "biopolitics" and both have been used to describe and explain the ways in which healthcare systems are (frequently) re-configured in advanced economies. Simply put, governmentality is the exercise of political power by the state but in conjunction with the active participation of the individual. Biopolitics refers to the exercise of political power over life.

The NHS in England offers a good illustration since, over the last 25 years, it has undergone considerable reorganization, both of secondary and primary care. To that end Fraser and colleagues (2019) have drawn on Foucault to examine the restructuring of services for stroke patients in London in 2011–12. They pose the question: "how can a biopolitical approach enhance understanding of major service change in healthcare?" (Fraser *et al.* 2019: 112). The reconfiguration of stroke services is considered as a biopolitical practice of security. The pre-existing services were regarded as inadequate (rather, in a state of crisis, putting people at risk). A plethora of evidence (including cartographic and statistical) was brought to bear to shed light on the geography of stroke incidence. The authors conclude that "major service change may be fruitfully conceptualized as a practice of security – a way of redefining a case, conceiving of risks and dangers, and averting crises in the interests of the population" (Fraser *et al.* 2019: 120).

Recall from above that various writers have suggested that "access" to health services means more than accessibility and availability – the dimensions that are most obviously geographical. But other dimensions, such as acceptability and adequacy, can be explored using post-structuralist (and social interactionist) approaches. A further approach that can be considered post-structuralist is non-representational theory (NRT). Andrews (2014) has considered its relevance in healthcare research, suggesting that it:

> could involve, for example, the unfolding of the space and time of a primary healthcare reception area and waiting room. People walking in, some sitting,

> others walking out, some coughing, doors opening and shutting, calls from staff that direct, phones ringing and computers bleeping, a television LED backlight flashing the daily news in the corner. (Andrews 2014: 166)

An NRT approach explores the atmospheres of interactions, particularly in everyday situations such as clinical settings. Whether NRT sheds any light on unequal access to healthcare is, however, unexamined.

Concluding remarks

This chapter has sought both to clarify what is meant by "access" to healthcare, and to introduce the variety of approaches that might be brought to bear on the subject.

We have seen that access can be conceived in terms of accessibility and that *spatial* accessibility has been, and continues to be, a key theme in our understanding of the geography of health services. This is a particular feature of what I have labelled "positivist" approaches. It is easy to criticize those studies that focus merely on spatial accessibility but it is clear that proximity to services is an important consideration in health-seeking behaviour. For example, children in South East Pennsylvania who live closer to an emergency department have greater use of those services while those living closer to a primary care provider make more use of those facilities (Ludwick *et al.* 2009).

I have sought to examine, and illustrate briefly, a variety of other approaches to the geography of healthcare services. Some of these seek explanations in terms of human agency, others more in terms of the structures that may determine healthcare utilization. Other, post-structuralist perspectives concern themselves more with affect and atmosphere: the day-to-day encounters with such facilities and their staff.

In terms of such approaches to studying access to healthcare there is clearly no "right" one and the choice depends very much on the question being posed. It would be foolish, as I noted elsewhere (Gatrell & Elliott 2015: 59–60), to try to shoehorn any particular study into a particular box. What matters more is whether empirical studies, a variety of which appear in this book, illuminate the subject they are concerned with. For example, if we are interested in how travel constrains or limits access we might require a survey of potential service users and try to quantify the different factors involved, perhaps with a view to generalizing this to other situations; this can be thought of as a positivist approach. If we were interested in the experiences of either travel to obtain healthcare or the ways in which people are "treated" there (less in terms of outcome and more in terms of the interactions they have with clinicians) then a social interactionist approach would have more value. We might be more concerned to reveal the organizational and structural determinants of care within a nation-state or regional context, in which case we might draw more on the insights from political economy.

If we think about *unequal* access to healthcare, where do the explanations lie? The decisions taken by (often anonymous) groups of people acting in and for global, national, regional and local organizations are crucial. But individual actors play a part too. For example, the more people seek private treatment, rather than that provided by a welfare state, the more systems themselves become privatized, giving an excuse for less investment in publicly funded services.

Geographers, particularly those concerned with economy, have debated at length the nature and importance of "scale" (Cresswell 2024: 218–21); the concept surely remains useful when discussing healthcare. If we think about seeking clinical care this is shaped by *local* service availability, by decisions taken by *regional* agencies, *nationally* (for example, how much government wants to allocate to healthcare funding) and *internationally* (by institutions such as the World Bank, especially in the Global South). The relative importance of these scales varies of course. In much of the Global North decisions taken by national governments are critical, while in many parts of the Global South spending on healthcare is constrained by structural adjustment policies imposed by the World Bank. The uptake, or lack thereof, of healthcare derives therefore from decisions made at the global, national, regional and local organizational levels.

It is time to consider how, and where, such decisions get made.

Further reading

Although they are over 15 years old the four chapters on "Health Care and Caring" in the collection edited by Brown *et al.* (2010) are excellent introductions to the literature on access to healthcare.

For a clearer understanding of how culture and place shape access to healthcare anything written by geographers Wil Gesler and Robin Kearns is worth reading. For a classic treatment see Gesler and Kearns (2002). For a commentary and reflections on the concept of the therapeutic landscape see Bell *et al.* (2018) and Kearns and Milligan (2020).

On landscapes of care, aside from work by Gesler and Kearns you will find work by Andrew Power, David Conradson, Janine Wiles and Christine Milligan of value. See for example: Milligan and Wiles (2010); Conradson (2003); Power (2008); and Power and Hall (2017).

References given in the text to "access" should be consulted but see also Carrillo *et al.* (2011) and the classic paper by Fiedler (1981). A thoughtful outline of different concepts of access to healthcare services is provided by Horrill *et al.* (2018). Another valuable contribution is Obrist *et al.* (2007). The classic geographical study of access to healthcare services is Joseph and Phillips (1984), while Curtis (2004) has chapters on landscapes of power, poverty and consumption. These are expanded on in Chapters 7 and 8 in Gatrell & Elliott (2015). On access to transgender healthcare, see Wright *et al.* (2021).

The International Journal of Health Geographics is a valuable source of material on measuring spatial accessibility to healthcare facilities.

For a clear, contemporary account of the various perspectives that geographers bring to bear on subject matter, I cannot recommend too highly Cresswell (2024). More specifically, and with regard to geographies of health, Gatrell & Elliott (2015) review in some detail the nature of the five broad perspectives covered above and give some examples of each.

3

THE POLITICAL ECONOMY OF HEALTHCARE SYSTEMS

> We witness people disillusioned by the commercial reorientation which sees patients recast as customers and a general striving to reclaim health as a quality less commodified, less medicalized and more connected to everyday life experiences. Gesler and Kearns (2002: 8)

A structuralist approach to healthcare was introduced briefly in the previous chapter. As an aspect of this a political economy perspective examines the impact on such care of how services are produced, distributed and consumed. What, it asks, are the political, economic and social contexts that shape the management, provision and utilization of care in a health system?

The chapter begins by examining the global picture of spending on healthcare, before offering a simple typology of healthcare systems and describing each of the four main models it comprises. Particular attention is then given to the US healthcare system, followed by some reflections on the spatial organization of healthcare systems. As part of a critical political economy focus I then say more about neoliberalism, austerity programmes and the growth of the private sector in different systems. The issue of provision for Indigenous populations merits particular attention, and the chapter concludes with a focus on colonialism and the decolonization of healthcare. First, however, having mentioned healthcare "systems" we need to unpack that term.

According to the World Health Organization (WHO) a health system refers to the set of all institutions, processes, resources and people that oversee and help improve health. "It manages the relationships between different actors and stakeholders involved in healthcare, including government agencies, healthcare providers, patients and their families, people and communities, civil society organizations and private sector entities".[1] This definition includes the role both of "government agencies" and "private sector

1. www.who.int/health-topics/health-systems-governance#tab=tab_1

entities" (along with others). The WHO goes on to assert that "effective health systems governance is essential for ensuring that healthcare services are accessible, equitable, efficient, affordable and of high quality for all". Note that access and equity feature explicitly in the WHO mantra. Whether equity and "high quality for all" are aligned with a role for "private sector entities" is a matter for debate. For some, healthcare is a "right" while for others it is a "commodity" (Box 3.1).

BOX 3.1 HEALTHCARE: COMMODITY OR A RIGHT?

The World Health Organization states: "The *right* to health for all people means that *everyone should have access to the health services they need*, when and where they need them, without suffering financial hardship"[2] (my emphasis). In an opposing view, Mark J. Perry, Senior Research Fellow at the American Enterprise Institute wrote in January 2017 that "medical care is a commodity, and treating it otherwise is foolhardy. Markets are the solution in medical care, just as they are in virtually every other area".[3]

There are many writers who subscribe to a rights-based approach, just as there are others aligned with a commodity-based approach that argues healthcare is a privilege and not a right. Christiansen (2017: 98) argues that "an optimal rights-based healthcare system would be publicly funded, provide universal coverage, and would be human resource-centred, with an emphasis on primary care". The late doctor-anthropologist Paul Farmer sought to put this into practice by establishing Partners in Health, whose mantra is "quality health care is a universal human right".

Commodification of healthcare occurs in various guises. It can include:

- the promotion of private insurance that supplements state provision;
- the supply and support of care by commercial enterprises (for example, through outsourcing activities in hospitals, including cleaning, catering and imaging);
- private investment in healthcare services (public–private partnerships);
- creating markets for different medical and healthcare products.

We see examples below in a discussion of the UK and US healthcare systems. Anticipating this, we note in particular that the latter is highly commodified, with corporate profits seeming to matter more than equal access to healthcare.

---

2. www.who.int/news-room/commentaries/detail/health-is-a-fundamental-human-right
3. www.aei.org/carpe-diem/health-care-is-a-commodity-not-a-right-and-markets-not-government-are-the-solution-in-medical-care/

Healthcare spending: the global picture

Spending on the consumption of healthcare (including all forms: primary and secondary) comes from a variety of sources: a mix of "domestic public" (government schemes and compulsory health insurance), "domestic private" (compulsory private and voluntary health insurance via employment) and out-of-pocket payments. Figure 3.1 shows the relationship between the main funding sources and financing schemes.

Figure 3.2 maps the global distribution of health expenditure as a proportion of gross domestic product (GDP). In countries of western Europe, the percentage of GDP spent on all healthcare in 2021 hovered around 10–13 per cent. In Canada and Australia, the figures were 12.3 per cent and 10.5 per cent respectively, while in the US it was 17.4 per cent.[4] The Health Foundation has argued that international comparisons are problematic. "While spend as a share of GDP is indicative of the priority countries attach to health, it reveals as much about a country's economy as it does about its health system".[5]

How does such expenditure translate into service provision, for example those engaged in delivering healthcare? There are, predictably, wide variations in the clinical workforce. Table 3.1 shows, for selected countries, data for the number of doctors, nurses

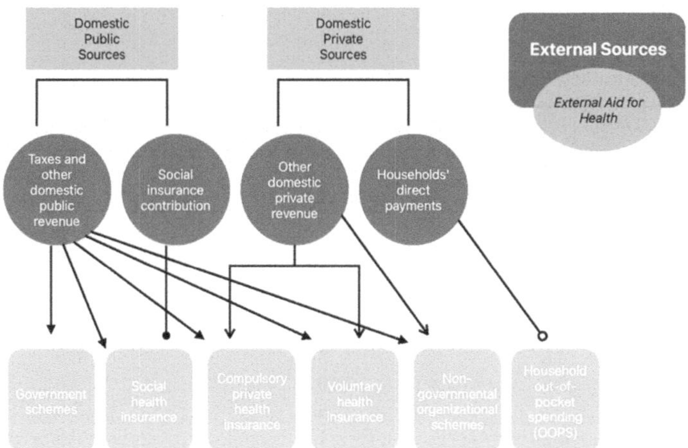

Figure 3.1 Relationship between main funding streams and financing schemes in health
Source: World Health Organization (2024).

4. https://ourworldindata.org/financing-healthcare
5. www.health.org.uk/publications/long-reads/the-complexities-of-using-international-comparisons-to-guide-nhs-reform

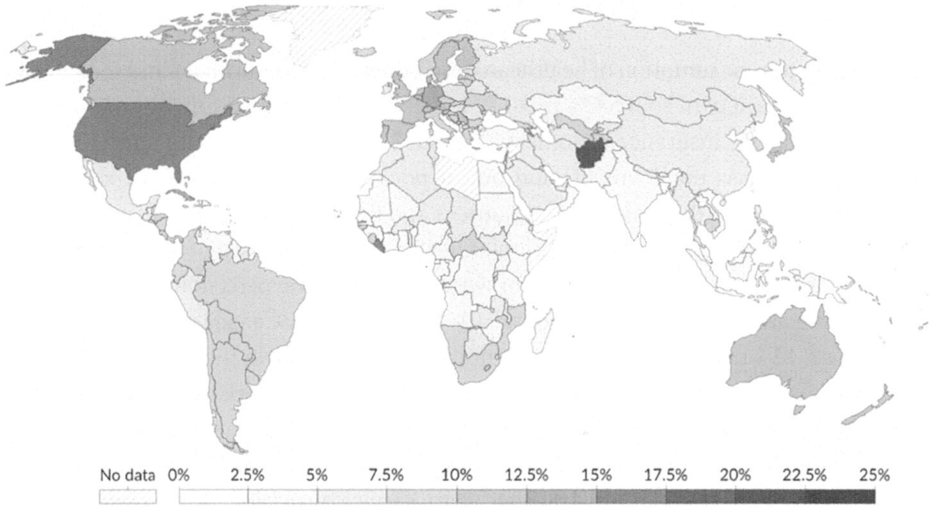

Figure 3.2 Total healthcare expenditure as a percentage of GDP (2021)
Source: https://ourworldindata.org/financing-healthcare

Table 3.1 Workforce data for selected countries (2024)

Country	*Doctors per 1,000*	*Nurses/midwives per 1,000*	*Hospital beds per 1,000*
Cuba	9.4	7.6	5.2
Germany	4.5	12.3	7.9
Australia	4.0	13.7	3.8
United States	3.6	11.9	2.8
New Zealand	3.6	11.7	2.5
France	3.3	9.4	5.8
UK	3.2	9.2	2.5
China	2.5	3.6	6.9
Canada	2.5	10.3	2.5
Brazil	2.1	5.5	2.5
India	0.7	1.7	0.5
Nigeria	0.4	1.7	0.9
Afghanistan	0.3	0.5	0.4
Democratic Republic of the Congo	0.2	1.2	0.8
Rwanda	0.1	0.9	0.1
Mozambique	0.1	0.5	0.1

Source: World Population Review.

and midwives, and the number of hospital beds per 1,000 people. All these figures are of course crude indicators, with numbers changing from year to year. Cuba – heading the table in terms of doctors – has a healthcare system (and its workforce) that is fully controlled by the government (Box 3.2). Data from the World Bank suggest that, in 2021, the country's domestic health expenditure per capita was US$2,778, well ahead of the second highest in Latin America (Uruguay: $1,736). Note that the UK lies well behind other Organisation for Economic Co-operation and Development (OECD) countries.

BOX 3.2 THE HEALTH SYSTEM IN CUBA

While Che Guevara is best known for his involvement in the Cuban revolution led by Fidel Castro in 1959, fewer will know him as a trained doctor who sought "to provide public health services for the greatest possible number of persons" (Bragg 2012: 11). Cuba's constitution commits to providing free medical and dental care to the entire population and prioritizing public health interventions. Community-based polyclinics, established in 1974, provide primary care (including maternity and child healthcare services), with a clear focus on the social determinants of health. In a very positive account, Keck and Reed (2012: e17) write:

> Few can match Cuba's record of 98% full immunization by the age of 2 years, vaccinating children against 13 illnesses; antenatal care for 95% of pregnant women by the end of their first trimester with rates of infant mortality less than 5 per 1000 births; and chronic disease control, including at least yearly blood pressure measurements for almost the entire population.

Further, evidence suggests that unlike countries in the Global North there is no inequality gradient in health outcomes according to socio-economic status (Nie *et al.* 2020). Although highly improbable, "the United States might also learn from Cuba's NHS and apply some of its principles to this country's market-driven health care system" (Keck & Reed 2012: e19).

Keck and Reed go on to suggest that the Cuban model of medical education aims to recruit medical students from communities in which they were born, and to have them work there after graduation. Yet as well as addressing domestic needs for medical professionals, Cuba has over 35,000 doctors working in countries in the Global South. This appears to come at a cost. Human Rights Watch reported in 2020 that Cuba's government regulations are such that doctors working abroad are subject to sanctions if they develop relationships with people who hold "hostile or contrary views to the Cuban revolution".[6] A report in 2019 suggested that almost half of doctors working abroad had their passports

6. www.hrw.org/news/2020/07/23/cuba-repressive-rules-doctors-working-abroad

confiscated by Cuban officials on their arrival overseas.[7] The *Harvard International Review* has called this "medical servitude".[8]

Not all authors share the rosy picture of healthcare in Cuba that is usually painted. For example, Gómez-Dantés (2018: 761) writes that:

> the Cuban health system is not performing as well as many believe: major progress in health status is limited to a few conditions, it lacks transparency and accountability, and its health policies have been implemented with little concern for certain basic rights. In sum, it is hardly a model to follow.

A typology of healthcare systems

Attempts to classify how healthcare systems are organized (and, crucially, funded) is fraught with difficulty since most countries have a mix of public and private provision. Furthermore, the nature and details of such systems change from time to time as new governments emerge.

Particular attention is paid below to the balance (or imbalance) between the role played by the state or government ("collectivist" provision) and that given over to private sector or market forces ("anti-collectivist" provision). Collectivist provision puts the community or society at the forefront of healthcare, whereas an anti-collectivist view prioritizes personal responsibility and the individual's right to choose (and maybe purchase) healthcare.

A simple classification of health systems operating across the world (taken from Physicians for a National Health Program[9]) distinguishes four such types: Beveridge; Bismarckian; national health insurance; and out-of-pocket. Each of these is discussed in turn.

The Beveridge healthcare system

The "Beveridge" system gets its name from William Beveridge, the British social economist whose report in 1942 set a blueprint for the establishment of the National Health Service (NHS) in the UK. In the Beveridge model, funding is mainly from general taxation and compulsory health insurance. The system comprises a centrally organized service with

7. www.bbc.co.uk/news/uk-48214513
8. https://hir.harvard.edu/medical-servitude-the-other-side-of-cuban-medical-diplomacy/
9. www.pnhp.org

provision mostly by publicly funded health providers (for primary care: family doctors or GPs; for secondary care: hospitals). In the UK, NHS structures differ according to whether we are concerned with England, Wales, Scotland, or Northern Ireland; most of what follows is based on the English context.

Over the past 25 years there has been a bewildering array of organizations that commission and deliver healthcare in England, reflecting decisions made by successive governments. Rather than rehearsing all these (see Baggott 2004 for an overview of some post-war changes) the most recent and significant incarnation of planning and commissioning bodies in England comprises integrated care boards (ICBs). An example is given in Box 3.3. Funding and decision-making are decentralized from the national government to regional bodies (the issue of decentralization is considered more fully later). ICBs fund healthcare, including that for hospitals. When – as is invariably the case – ICBs are required by national government to make annual savings, they pass these over to hospitals, meaning fewer staff, less on maintenance and so on.

Geography matters, since different ICBs can adopt different policies. For example, if in vitro fertilization (IVF) is requested, the number of cycles that are funded depends where you live. In 2025 most ICBs, like Lancashire and South Cumbria (see Box 3.3), offered just one. But in the adjacent ICB (North East and North Cumbria) you could potentially access three rounds if required. Where you live within the county of Cumbria makes a big difference. The same is true in the East Midlands of the UK where different ICBs have different policies. Dr Dave Briggs from Nottinghamshire ICB (permitting only one cycle of IVF) says: "*That doesn't mean to say that we don't recognise the importance of IVF and fertility services but we also need to ensure that delivers within our financial means and also a lot of other services at the same time*".[10] This decentralization creates what are called "postcode lotteries". Of course, the private sector is always available – £9,000 per cycle – if it is affordable. But this is *potential* access and, as we see throughout this book, *realized* access depends on location relative to clinic availability. Jones *et al.* (2023) illustrate this clearly, finding that geographical accessibility to clinics providing assisted reproduction is significantly lower in the poorest and most deprived areas in England. We see that geography matters both in terms of what is potentially offered and what is realistically accessible in terms of travel time.

ICBs link up with local government authorities and other partners to form integrated care systems (ICSs), which, in theory, help link health services and social care. The government allocates funding to ICSs using a formula based on "a complex assessment of factors such as demography, morbidity, deprivation, and the unavoidable cost of providing services in different areas". This is supposed "to make geographic distribution fair and objective, so that it more clearly reflects local healthcare need and helps to reduce

10. https://www.bbc.co.uk/news/articles/ckglq7kn11jo

BOX 3.3 AN INTEGRATED CARE BOARD IN ENGLAND: LANCASHIRE AND SOUTH CUMBRIA

ICBs have a big job. Like others, my own local ICB (Lancashire and South Cumbria) has lofty aims:

> Our role as an ICB is to join up health and care services, improve people's health and wellbeing, and make sure everyone has the same access to services and gets the same outcomes from treatment. We also oversee how money is spent and make sure health services are working well and are of high quality.[11]

Workforce issues are a particular concern (and we return to this issue in Chapter 4). This particular ICB reports a shortage of staff, with vacancy rates that are above the national average (9 per cent versus 7 per cent). In addition, more than one-fifth of the clinical staff (8,000 people) are aged over 55 years and likely to be retiring relatively soon. "Alongside this, our ability to recruit is impacted by the condition of our infrastructure and the reputation and quality of our services". This is refreshingly honest, but it is hardly reassuring to prospective service users to hear that facilities are in a poor shape and that the services do not have a great reputation.

As noted earlier, governments often refashion health organizations. In April 2026 some ICBs merged into "clusters".[12]

health inequalities".[13] Whether these aims are being met is a moot point. Certainly, general practitioners (GPs) do not feel that the funding is equitable, with their professional organization (Royal College of General Practitioners, RCGP) arguing that the funding does not allow adequately for levels of deprivation among the populations they serve. As the Chair of the RCGP put it: "*GPs and their teams across the country are dealing with intense resource and workforce pressures – but this is being felt more acutely in more economically deprived areas. Where people live shouldn't dictate the care they have access to and receive*".[14]

11. www.lancashireandsouthcumbria.icb.nhs.uk/
12. https://www.england.nhs.uk/integratedcare/integrated-care-in-your-area/more-about-each-integrated-care-system/
13. www.england.nhs.uk/wp-content/uploads/2019/05/allocations-2019-20-technical-guide-to-formulae-v1.2.pdf
14. https://www.theguardian.com/politics/article/2024/may/22/doctors-call-for-funding-reform-to-tackle-health-disparities-across-england-royal-college-of-gps

The concerns of the RCGP have to be taken seriously, since the vast majority of healthcare takes place in the primary care setting, not the hospital. For example, in 2021/22 there were 320 million GP appointments in England, compared with 122 million hospital outpatient appointments and 24.4 million attendances at A&E.[15] It is for these reasons that here, and in the following chapter, considerable attention is given to primary care.

The Bismarck healthcare system

The Bismarck scheme is a "mixed" model (using both public and private provision), funded mostly by mandatory insurance schemes which provide universal coverage. Examples are Germany (hence the scheme named after the former nineteenth-century Chancellor Otto von Bismarck), France, Austria, Switzerland and Japan.

In Germany health insurance is mandatory and comprises both statutory health insurance (SHI) known as "sickness funds", which covers almost 90 per cent of the population, and private health insurance. The SHI is not administered by the federal government; this has a regulatory, but not a provider role. This is much the same in France where the Ministry of Health has overall control and monitoring but regional health authorities are responsible for public health and healthcare planning and finance. Again, there is decentralization.

Some writers (notably, those on the political right) argue that the UK should move away from the tax-based NHS towards a statutory social health insurance model such as these. However, others suggest that:

> switching to an SHI system would be costly and disruptive, with no evidence it would deliver benefits. Instead, UK policymakers should recognize the strengths of the UK's existing model – low administrative costs and low financial barriers to care compared with other countries – and focus on how to secure long-term sustainable funding in the face of growing demand.[16]

The national health insurance system

The "national health insurance" system (see Table 3.1 for examples) has some features in common with the first two. Take Canada as an example. While the providers are from the private sector they are funded by a government insurance programme into

15. www.health.org.uk/publications/long-reads/the-complexities-of-using-international-comparisons-to-guide-nhs-reform
16. www.health.org.uk/publications/reports/is-the-grass-really-greener

which the public pays. Via the Canada Health Act the federal government sets national standards and provides finance to the provinces and territories which are given authority to organize and manage all primary and secondary healthcare based on regional needs (decentralization again). The Act provides for "medically necessary services" but these are not defined, leaving provinces and territories to make their own decisions. For example, if IVF is sought, Alberta and Saskatchewan, along with the territories, do not offer coverage, suggesting geographical inequity across the country.

Expenditure on healthcare varies considerably between provinces and territories. Nunavat, Yukon and the Northwest Territories (NWT) spend the most per capita, the first of these spending Ca$17,500 per capita in 2023, compared with Ca$5,340 in Ontario. Such differences are in large part due to the sparsity of population distribution, the network of health centres in small, remote communities and the travel costs in reaching them. The federal government provides direct funding to First Nations and Inuit people, including primary care and emergency services in remote areas that are otherwise unserved. However, during the period 2010–14 "the territorial governments [were] still the main source of healthcare financing, accounting for 66%, 69% and 80% of total health expenditures in Yukon, NWT and Nunavut, respectively. Direct federal health expenditures did not exceed 15% in any of the three territories" (Young *et al.* 2016: 63).

We consider later the support given to First Nations and Inuit Canadians, as well as other Indigenous populations.

Out-of-pocket healthcare

In many countries of the Global South there is no national healthcare system or universal coverage and people pay "out of pocket" (Figure 3.3). Access to providers is limited and depends on ability to pay. The proportion of such payments as a total of all healthcare expenditure in a country is 75 per cent in Nigeria and 77 per cent in Afghanistan; in the latter, the burden lies heavily on women in particular (Box 3.4). However, in some countries (for example, Mozambique and Zambia) the proportion of out-of-pocket expenditure is significantly lower.

Not included in the four-fold classification outlined above is a private insurance model of the form found in the US, although as we see below that country has some social provision in the form of Medicare and Medicaid. The American pressure group "Physicians for a National Health Program" has more to say about all four systems considered above and offers a pithy summary, as follows:

> These four models should be fairly easy for Americans to understand because we have elements of all of them in our fragmented national healthcare apparatus. When it comes to treating veterans, we're Britain or Cuba. For Americans

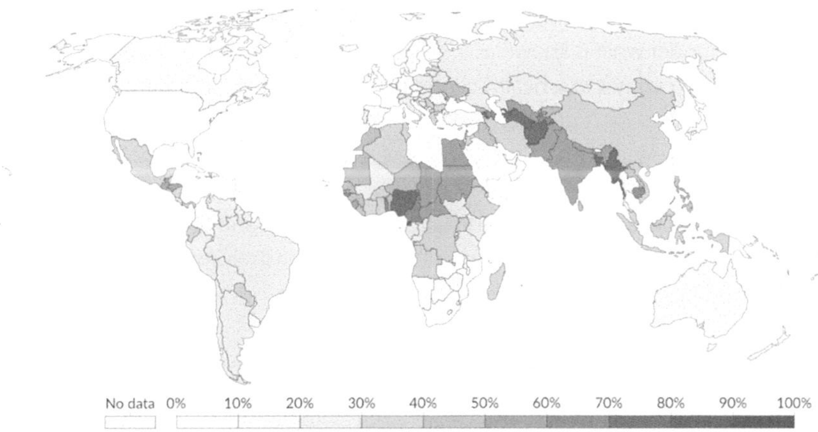

Figure 3.3 Share of out-of-pocket expenditure on healthcare in 2021
Source: https://ourworldindata.org/financing-healthcare

BOX 3.4 THE COSTS OF HEALTHCARE IN AFGHANISTAN

The charity Médecins Sans Frontières (MSF, Doctors without Borders) describes Afghanistan's healthcare system as "dysfunctional", noting in 2023 that the humanitarian crisis in the country was in part due to the poor treatment of women. Declining incomes and international sanctions mean that respondents in the MSF survey found themselves declining or delaying medical care because they could not afford it. As Marieh explained, after arriving at the MSF-supported Herat Regional Hospital:

> *When my child was sick, we went to one of the private clinics and received a prescription for drugs that cost 1,000 AFG* [around US$16]. *They didn't help. We also tried a nearby public hospital, but doctors there gave us only half a tablet, not all the medication* [we needed] ... *Now we're here. My baby is worse, and I owe a lot of money we borrowed for transport.*

MSF's country representative explained that:

> One of the main problems in Afghanistan is that peripheral health facilities are neither well-equipped, adequately resourced nor properly staffed. This means people in rural areas need to travel vast distances for quality treatment, even though they often cannot afford such journeys without plunging themselves into debt.

Women are particularly constrained in their movement to access healthcare, since they are required (under what is known as "*mahram*") to be accompanied by a male relative. Even when they can get to a health centre the staff find that: "sometimes mothers are so malnourished they can't produce milk for their children. We see them putting tea in bottles to give to new-born babies of only seven or eight days, which can be very dangerous".[17]

In a recent review of healthcare under the Taliban, Basij-Rasikh and colleagues (2024: 6) quote a woman doctor who paints a depressing picture of the likely future of the female healthcare workforce:

> *The first big challenge is that we don't want to be the last generation of female doctors. We need another generation to come to study to develop and become female doctors. When schools are closed, when girls couldn't even go to the school, how can I be hopeful that when I become retired, when I become old, there will be another female doctor to provide help for a female?*

It is worth referring back to the story of Nurse Sadia Khan told in Chapter 1.

---

over the age of 65 on Medicare, we're Canada. For working Americans who get insurance on the job, we're Germany. For the 15 percent of the population who have no health insurance, the United States is Cambodia or Burkina Faso.[18]

The US healthcare system

The key issue in the US healthcare system is which, and how, people are insured for healthcare. Insurance can be private (self-funded, or paid for by employers) or public. The latter include Medicare and Medicaid (Box 3.5). The percentage of the population insured privately in 2022 was 65.6 while for Medicare and Medicaid it was 18.7 and 18.8 respectively. Across the US as a whole, 8 per cent of the population was uninsured in 2022, down from 15 per cent in 2012 as a result of the Affordable Care Act (ACA) that

17. The quotes in Box 3.4 are from www.doctorswithoutborders.ca/afghanistan-deprived-of-healthcare-by-poverty-restrictions-and-a-disfunctional-system/
18. www.pnhp.org/single_payer_resources/health_care_systems_four_basic_models.php

was introduced by President Obama (hence it is sometimes referred to as "Obamacare"). Lack of insurance is socially and spatially patterned. In 2022 16.8 per cent of the Hispanic population and 8.7 per cent of the Black population was uninsured, compared with 5.3 per cent of the white population.[19] There is a clear geography to this (Figure 3.4): in 2024 about 17 per cent in Texas were uninsured, 11 per cent in Florida and Wyoming, but only 3 per cent in Massachusetts.

Lack of insurance has an impact on access to preventive healthcare and treatment for chronic disease and acute episodes. Even with insurance the costs of care are prohibitive. Christiansen (2017) reports a comparative study of healthcare systems of high-income countries which suggested that 39 per cent of people surveyed in the US who had a medical problem did not seek care because of the high cost, compared with only 1 per cent in the UK.

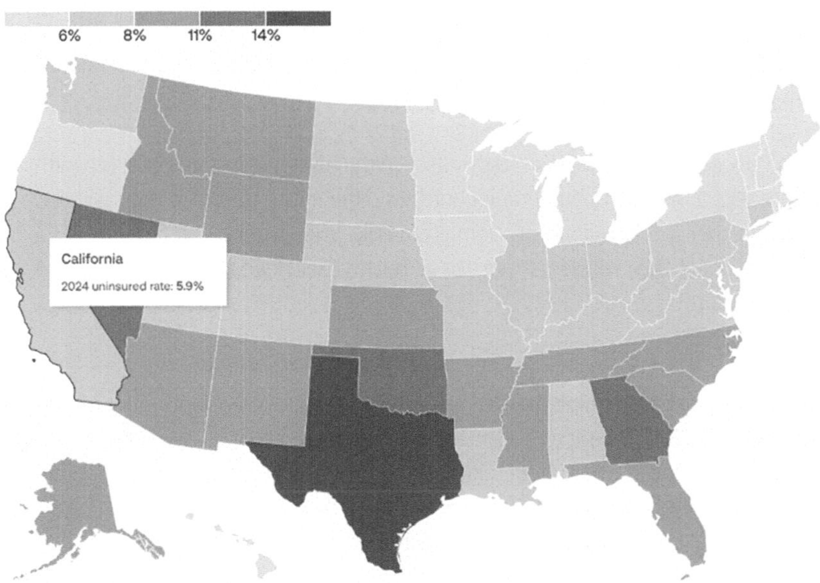

Figure 3.4 Percentage of the total population in the US that is uninsured (2024)
Source: www.usafacts.org

19. Peter G. Peterson Foundation: www.pgpf.org

BOX 3.5 MEDICARE AND MEDICAID

Established in 1965, Medicaid provides health coverage to families and individuals (adults, children, people with disabilities) on low incomes. Although a federal programme, it is also funded by states and these have discretion as to the level of funding they provide. Not all states implemented an expansion of Medicaid funding when the government introduced this in 2020 as part of the Affordable Care Act. As of 2021 37 states expanded Medicaid coverage but 12 (mostly in the Deep South) opted not to. This has consequences for child health, evidence suggesting that children with Medicaid coverage have better educational outcomes and better health.[20] Medicaid expansion has also been associated with earlier diagnosis of breast cancer among low-income women, because of increased uptake of screening, as suggested by a geographical study in Ohio (Dong *et al.* 2022).

Medicare funds those aged over 65 years, but also some people with disabilities. Within Medicare there are options to take out additional private insurance ("Medicare Advantage" and "Medigap") and there is a geography to this, with plans depending on state, county and even zip code. Some people are eligible for both Medicare and Medicaid.

For a fuller description of the US healthcare system in 2024 see the Professional Society for Health Economics and Outcomes Research website.[21] To set this in an international context see also a report by the Commonwealth Fund in 2024.[22] This looked at health system performance in 10 countries, noting that:

> The U.S. continues to be in a class by itself in the underperformance of its health care sector. While the other nine countries differ in the details of their systems and in their performance on domains, unlike the U.S. they all have found a way to meet their residents' most basic health care needs, including universal coverage.

In terms of access to healthcare the Netherlands ranked top and the US bottom.

Readers should bear in mind that, following the election of President Trump for a second term starting in 2025, the picture painted in this section may well be dated. At the time of writing his so-called "One Big Beautiful Bill" promises to increase Medicare premiums as well as increasing employer-sponsored insurance costs. Some writers suggest that the impact will be felt particularly acutely by Black people.[23]

20. www.cbpp.org/research/policy-basics-introduction-to-medicaid
21. www.ispor.org/heor-resources/more-heor-resources/us-healthcare-system-overview/us-healthcare-system-overview-background-page-1
22. www.commonwealthfund.org/publications/fund-reports/2024/sep/mirror-mirror-2024
23. www.naacpldf.org/case-issue/trumps-one-big-beautiful-bill-act-explained/

Aside from considering who the uninsured population are and where they live, there are other issues concerning structural change in the health insurance industry: specifically, the merging of insurance companies, which have formed monopolies that can limit consumer choice and keep premiums high. This is part of a wider hijacking of healthcare by corporate capitalism (Box 3.6). "The healthcare industry, like other sectors of the economy, has increasingly experienced domination by fewer and fewer, larger and larger corporations; this is true for health insurance companies, medical providers, and pharmaceutical companies" (Perry & Bernasek 2024: 3).

BOX 3.6 MONOPOLY POWER IN THE US HEALTHCARE SYSTEM: THE EXAMPLE OF PARKVIEW HEALTH

Centred on Fort Wayne in Indiana, Parkview Health is a very large health system that serves a population of over 1.3 million people living in north-east Indiana and north-west Ohio. According to its website "Parkview Health is the region's largest employer, with 16,000 co-workers at 14 hospitals and more than 200 outpatient centers and physician offices".[24] Its focus is the Regional Medical Center (Figure 3.5) known by some employees as "Emerald City" for its "ritzy amenities and green corporate branding".

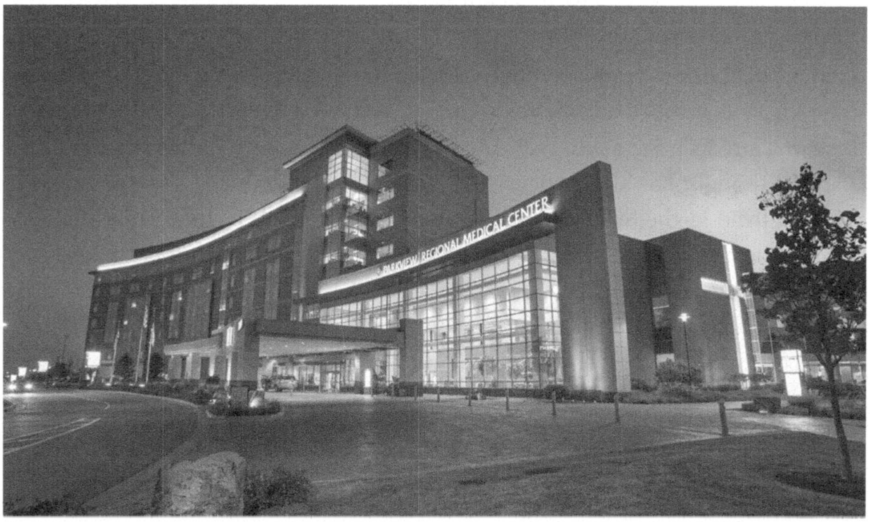

Figure 3.5 Parkview Health's Regional Medical Center
Source: www.parkview.com/locations/parkview-regional-medical-center

24. https://www.parkview.com/about-us

In a critical article by the UK's *Guardian* newspaper it is claimed that Parkview dominates the regional healthcare market and sets high prices for care and treatment. "This consolidation, former employees say, has allowed Parkview to control referral flows, routing primary care patients to their own costly specialists and facilities, even if those patients could get the same services elsewhere for less". Parkview employees confirm that doctors are ranked according to the patients they refer on to other Parkview hospitals, with remuneration and bonuses given according to patient volume and referrals for costly procedures. "Revenue pressure was even brought down to the level of nurses – some of whom say they have been pushed to charge for the smallest of items from Kleenexes to batteries". A charge of almost $400 was made for putting a small sticking plaster onto a girl's finger – taking all of 10 seconds. It costs rather more to be transferred to the hospital following a major road accident, as uninsured Tom Frost discovered when presented with a bill for $629,386.50. An independent auditor thought less than half of this was reasonable.[25]

There are many stories told by American citizens who live abroad and have had very different experiences of care and treatment compared with what they would have encountered back home. Unlike some people who travel abroad specifically to receive healthcare (see pp. 154–7), others have moved overseas, either for work or family reasons. The following is a compelling illustration:

> I am a U.S. Citizen living abroad in Canada for almost two decades. Over that time I have developed a tremendous appreciation for the Canadian Healthcare system. I am deeply grateful that when I am ill, or a family member has been ill, the first thought has always been to get the appropriate, necessary treatment. When I lived in the States I lived through many periods of time with little or no healthcare. I would suffer unnecessarily to avoid the cost of care. Like so many Americans I thought I had to "be stoic" to avoid going into debt as "just a part of life." I no longer live with this fear in Canada. I have witnessed elderly friends admitted to very good nursing home facilities they could never afford in the States that are completely covered by the Canadian government. I have witnessed people treated with dignity regardless of their ability to pay. I have experienced recuperating from illness and injury without the fear and dread of the many "surprise" bills that will soon arrive in the mail. So my "healthcare story" is this: the Canadian Healthcare system – just by its very existence – has brought incalculable reassuring comfort and peace for my future into my life.[26]

25. Source, including direct quotes, www.theguardian.com/us-news/2024/oct/17/indiana-medical-debt-parkview-hospital
26. www.democratsabroad.org/healthcare_stories

This vignette tells us vividly that accessing healthcare in the US for some depends upon cost. And the affordability of healthcare may be shaped by corporate power.

There are some in the US who seek to adopt a Beveridge-like healthcare system: a "publicly financed, non-profit, single-payer national health program that would fully cover medical care for all Americans". This is the stated view of Physicians for a National Health Program, supported by Democratic Senator Bernie Sanders. Such an aspiration is unlikely to bear fruit given the Trump presidency.

Organizing healthcare services

I want in this section to say something about the spatial organization of healthcare services. First, I consider the trade-off between efficiency and equity. I then examine the issue of decentralizing healthcare: the spatial level at which responsibility for delivery is conferred.

It goes without saying that healthcare services should be offered that are effective and confer health benefits. But for those authorities providing them there will be an interest in providing them "efficiently", in the sense of maximizing utility (health benefit) while minimizing cost to the healthcare system. Consumers too are interested in maximizing health benefit but are likely to be more interested in minimizing the cost of access or travel. Both providers and consumers should wish to provide services equitably and this means locating services that are geographically accessible to consumers and particularly to those in greatest need.

More concretely, looking at the provision of both primary and secondary (hospital) care, while it may be more cost-effective to operate a smaller number of large centres (where there are likely to be economies of scale), these may not meet the criterion of equity, since service users will inevitably have further to travel. Set against that, however, is the possibility that larger centres may have a wider range of expertise and have a great volume of activity, counteracting the distances to be overcome. While that provision may seem "unjust" the potential concentration of clinical expertise can outweigh the costs of travel.

As noted above (pp. 11–15), for the consumer this is hardly an abstract exercise. Would one prefer to incur greater costs of travel and hospital stay in order to be treated in a specialist centre that is likely to have undertaken numerous similar procedures to the one that is needed? Such a preference may not be available to a poorer consumer worried about extra costs of transport, suggesting there are clear issues of equity.

In the US there is considerable evidence that fewer, larger hospitals – in effect, a regionalization of access – result in better outcomes for patients. Yet evidence from surveys of prospective patients suggest there are likely to be barriers to such regionalization, including transport constraints and the lack of social/family support, felt particularly by older people, which would be provided more locally (see, e.g., Symer *et al.* 2019). Research comparing outcomes at centres providing low and high volumes of surgery suggests that while the latter leads to better outcomes (such as lower mortality rates, shorter length of stay) there were inequities in that high-volume hospitals seem to treat lower proportions of non-white and female patients, as well as those treated under Medicaid (Williamson *et al.* 2023).

Having considered the relative advantages and disadvantages of geographical rationalization of healthcare services – whether to concentrate or "centralize" services or to provide large numbers of smaller facilities as a kind of dispersed or "decentralized" configuration – I look now at a different meaning of decentralization. This is the transfer of responsibility, whether political, organizational or financial (or all three) from the level of the national government to lower (regional or local) levels within a country. At what geographic scale (national, regional, local) should health services be managed and funded? Should healthcare planning, operation and decision-making be transferred from the state to lower organizational levels?

The Alma Ata declaration in 1978 that gave an impetus to primary care was quite explicit about the need for decentralization. It wrote:

> The general administrative system of a country is important for ensuring coordinated contributions to development from the different sectors concerned. In the past, there has been a tendency to concentrate almost entirely on the central administrative level. *Only recently has attention been focused on local levels. The importance of decentralization to intermediate levels, such as provincial or district levels, now has to be stressed.* These levels are near enough to communities to respond sensitively to their practical problems and needs.[27]

Decentralization is, for some writers, a term with multiple dimensions. As Winchester and King (2018: 200) put it: "decentralization is a multifaceted and multisectoral process that has the potential, over time, to rectify historical inequality by empowering local administrative units to control their own healthcare agendas and resources with the intention of tailoring service provision to the local population". Yet what is being transferred from the "centre" to the "periphery"? Is it political, administrative, financial control or some combination of all three? And what evidence is there that inequality is reduced? Certainly, in a rural South African context Winchester and King (2018: 201) note that, despite decentralization of healthcare "the landscapes of healthcare remain uneven".

Political decentralization (devolution) means transferring governance to lower level authorities. Following Rotulo *et al.* (2002) economic decentralization can mean one of two things: fiscal federalism or fiscal decentralization. In the former, healthcare resources are pooled centrally and then distributed to regional or local bodies who set their own

27. www.unicef.org/media/85611/file/Alma-Ata-conference-1978-report.pdf; reference is p. 51, my italics.

spending priorities. "Central governments can control their public healthcare expenditure and address regional heterogeneity by providing equitably tailored budgets" (Rotulo *et al.* 2002: 110). This is what happens in England as budgets are allocated to ICBs (pp. 39–41) according to a complex resource allocation formula that provides a degree of equitable funding. Fiscal decentralization means that local governments hold the purse strings. But this has equity implications if richer areas have more money to spend. In some countries (such as Spain) there is *political* decentralization but limited fiscal decentralization. Healthcare organization is devolved to the 17 autonomous communities but the finance is largely a central government matter. There are many reviews (e.g. Sapkota *et al.* 2023) that consider what impact decentralization (of various types) has on healthcare provision and equity. In Spain, "healthcare devolution has not led to an expansion of regional inequalities in healthcare outcomes and outputs" (Costa-Font & Rico 2006: 875).

Neoliberalism, austerity and the growth of the private sector

As we have seen, the role of private capital and the increased role played by monopoly power are key features of the US healthcare system. We considered briefly in the previous chapter the ways in which neoliberalism has shaped healthcare. The Marxist health services scholar Howard Waitzkin (2020) has done more than most to make explicit the impacts of this ideology. He suggests that "under Obamacare, the capitalist state has continued to prioritize protection of the capitalist economic system, in this case by overseeing huge subsidies for private insurance and pharmaceutical corporations" (Waitzkin 2020: 460). Little has changed since he wrote.

But the heavy hand of private capital is not restricted to the US. Göttems and Mollo (2020) explore the impacts of neoliberalism on health systems in Latin America and the Caribbean. Here, the loans made to countries by the World Bank and International Monetary Fund to relieve debt burdens went hand in hand with reductions in public spending, privatization and deregulation. The consequences included more cost-sharing ("co-payments") between the state and the "consumer", more private healthcare provision, decentralization of services away from the state to local government (with the poorest regions "punished"; Göttems & Mollo 2020: 6). These assertions echo those of Homedes and Ugalde (2005) who pay particular attention to Colombia and Chile. Even the Chilean Ministry of Health acknowledged that the Chilean health system was "extremely inequitable" (in Homedes & Ugalde 2005: 7). Private sector insurance companies see high profit margins as they can "cherry-pick" patients, often those who are wealthy and better educated. The authors are even more scathing about the Colombian healthcare system, noting that:

> the country has followed very closely the World Bank reform blueprints, [but] in spite of a very substantial increase in healthcare expenditures, a large percentage

> of the population continues to be uncovered, the poor continue to have difficulties in accessing services because of high co-payments, there are no measurable efficiency and medical care quality improvements, public healthcare has deteriorated, and health equity has suffered. (Homedes & Ugalde 2005: 9)

But this perspective is 20 years old and recent evidence suggests there are ongoing significant geographical variations in public healthcare between urban and rural areas. Those living in the cities (Bogota, Medellin and Cali) can access high quality care but in rural areas care is much more basic and, inevitably, there are long journey times to clinics and hospitals. As we see in Chapter 7, the large volume of refugees coming into the country from neighbouring Venezuela puts additional pressures on the Colombian healthcare system.

Benbow (2023) notes that, according to the WHO, privatization is "a process in which nongovernmental actors become increasingly involved in the financing and/or provision of healthcare services". He goes on to suggest that "this accurately describes what has been occurring within the English NHS" (Benbow 2023: 24), echoing Roderick and Pollock's (2022: 470) assertion that "England is now moving decisively toward a marketized, two-tier, mixed-funding system with several similarities to the United States". Goodair and Reeves (2022: e639) suggest that "evidence of the impact of so-called creeping privatization in general, and in the NHS in England in particular, remains uncertain", although their own empirical work illustrates that outsourcing to for-profit companies has worsened population health and increased mortality rates. Their wider review of privatization in high-income countries suggests a consistent picture of its negative impacts on healthcare (Goodair & Reeves 2024).

Regardless of the possible impacts of private sector healthcare it shows no sign of lessening, certainly in the UK. The NHS waiting list in England was 4.57 million in 2019 but had risen to 7.77 million in September 2023 before falling to 6.24 million in February 2025. This high volume has prompted the NHS to pay private hospitals to treat patients (paying £2.1 billion in 2023 to do so) but has also led to individuals to pay for their care in such hospitals, either using private insurance or their own pockets. The Health Foundation reported in 2022 that the volume of care outsourced to the private sector was 16 per cent, with the share of ophthalmic care (often, cataract surgery) amounting to 34 per cent. The overall shares vary regionally, from 7 per cent in London to 21 per cent in Yorkshire and they vary according to material deprivation, being 11 per cent in the most deprived areas to 25 per cent in the least deprived areas. Table 3.2 compares admissions (by UK region) to private hospitals that are paid for by insurance schemes or are self-funded. To some extent, as the table shows, this reflects the different levels of wealth in each region, as measured by GDP per capita.

Table 3.2 Admissions to, and funding of, private healthcare in UK regions and GDP per capita

	Admissions		
Region	*Insured*	*Self-pay*	*GDP per capita (£)*
London	54,340	13,810	57,338
South East	30,235	11,105	36,425
East England	18,085	7,150	30,218
North West	10,665	5,720	29,748
West Midlands	8,560	5,060	27,278
South West	8,380	7,325	30,188
East Midlands	6,085	3,305	26,755
Yorkshire & Humberside	5,850	4,185	27,649
North East	1,850	1,680	24,172
Scotland	6,255	4,900	30,586
Wales	3,090	4,250	24,443
Northern Ireland	2,710	2,415	26,480
Total	156,100	70,960	

Source: https://www.phin.org.uk/news/PHIN-Private-market-update-September-2023
Note: Private healthcare data are for first quarter of year, 2023. GDP data are for 2022.

As the Health Foundation observes, if the independent sector further increases the share of NHS-funded care it delivers, these findings raise questions about whether different areas of the country will have equal access to care.[28]

The American public intellectual Noam Chomsky (2011) has written that the "standard technique of privatization [is]: defund, make sure things don't work, people get angry, you hand it over to private capital". Others concur. "It needs to be emphasized that the under-financing of healthcare services by the State, which opens up opportunities for private enterprises, is often a deliberate ploy employed by States under the influence of neoliberal policies".[29] One such aspect of neoliberalism (the introduction of austerity programmes – a political economic choice) is discussed in Box 3.7.

Indigenous healthcare, colonialism and the decolonization of healthcare

In a chapter on the political economy of healthcare it is important to address whether such care is, or is not, provided to Indigenous populations (a personal story of which we

28. www.health.org.uk/reports-and-analysis/analysis/waiting-for-nhs-hospital-care-the-role-of-the-independent-sector
29. www.altersummit.eu/analyse/article/commodification-of-health-the-challenge-facing-health-systems

BOX 3.7 AUSTERITY AND ITS IMPACT ON HEALTHCARE

Memories can be short and it is easy to forget the impact that the global financial crisis of 2008 and subsequent budget cuts had on healthcare and equity of access. Austerity programmes – part of the neoliberal project – were introduced across much of Europe. Stuckler *et al.* (2017) argue that austerity has negative impacts on the social determinants of health (such as poverty and unemployment) but also in restricting access to healthcare. The latter is the focus here. Stuckler and colleagues noted that the largest cuts to health budgets were in Greece, Ireland, Latvia and Portugal.

A wide-ranging review (Doetsch *et al.* 2023) found that austerity programmes in the European Union led to healthcare needs being unmet and a reduction in healthcare utilization. Unmet needs are defined as "the differences, if any, between those services judged necessary to deal appropriately with defined health problems and those services actually being received" (Zavras *et al.* 2016: 2). Within particular countries there were regional differences in healthcare provision and utilization. In Italy, for example, between 2006 and 2015 while there was no change in the frequency of visits to doctors in the (wealthier) northern region, the (poorer) south of the country saw such visits falling by a third. In Spain, access to care was impacted by a reduction in the number of beds and poorer availability of out-of-hours emergency care in rural areas. Further, cuts that were imposed by austerity measures in Spain led to more self-medication, increased visits to accident and emergency facilities and longer waiting times for GP appointments. Across much of Europe the impacts were not felt equally: "vulnerable populations were more affected by the implemented austerity measures than the general population regarding their access to care" (Doetsch *et al.* 2023: 9).

In Greece the government was forced by a combination of the European Commission, the European Central Bank and the International Monetary Fund into signing an "Economic Adjustment Programme" that required tax increases and reductions in wages and pensions. Statistical analysis by Zavras *et al.* (2016) using national survey data revealed that financial reasons were responsible for a far higher proportion of them having unmet needs in 2011 than in 2006. Survey participants in the lowest income group in need of medical care were 2.65 times more likely to see those needs unmet compared with people in the next highest income group.

In England, the Nuffield Trust reported in 2023 that restricted funding for NHS hospitals left them without the means "to recruit adequate numbers of staff or invest in its disintegrating estate and equipment", forcing them into:

> having to make a series of short-term, often self-defeating savings to balance the books … propped up only through haphazard emergency injections of

> extra cash. This spared the NHS from the sort of total financial collapse seen in the public health system in Greece from 2010.[30]

The Nuffield Trust also referred to "woeful workforce planning" that included cuts in the number of training places for nurses, although recent data suggest that there has been a significant increase in the number of nurses employed since 2015 (set against a loss of about 2,000 GPs).[31] This is explored further in Chapter 4.

---

saw in Chapter 1). We also need to discuss provision under colonialism and attempts to decolonize healthcare.

It is possible here only to scratch the surface of how, where and why colonial powers developed health services during the nineteenth and early twentieth centuries. Briefly, resources were directed more to settler rather than Indigenous populations. As Farmer (2020: 252) puts it: "colonial efforts to provide health services were ... paltry". Little had changed during the first part of the twenty-first century. Farmer's book, dealing with Ebola in West Africa in particular, emphasizes that more attention was given to containing disease spread than providing healthcare for those infected. In an important paper on South Africa Winchester and King (2018) argue that even after the abolition of apartheid the country continues to suffer the impacts of colonial and apartheid policies that sought to benefit the white minority population. As they put it: "historical systems of spatial segregation also shaped unequal healthcare structures, services, expenditures, and accessibility across the country" (Winchester & King 2018: 202). Expenditure was used to cement racial domination by the white population. Post-apartheid, little has changed. "Poorer, rural, and black African populations face barriers of distance, transportation, and lack of adequate services at healthcare facilities" (Winchester & King 2018: 202).

Access to healthcare in Israel (and Gaza) is also instructive. Included in the Declaration of the Establishment of the State of Israel in 1948 was the statement that "it will ensure complete equality of social and political rights to all its inhabitants irrespective of religion, race or sex". To what extent has this "equality" been extended to Palestinians living in Israel and the occupied territories (notably, Gaza)? A recent review from the Center for Human Rights at Harvard University suggests that the Palestinian population living within Israel has poorer outcomes than the Jewish population, an observation confirmed by the Israeli Ministry of Health (Tanous *et al.* 2023). Tanous and colleagues suggest that health inequalities among Palestinians are rooted in structural racism, reflecting a "settler

30. www.nuffieldtrust.org.uk/news-item/what-was-austeritys-toll-on-the-nhs-before-the-pandemic
31. See: www.nuffieldtrust.org.uk/resource/the-nhs-workforce-in-numbers.

colonialism" where the "impacts of settler colonialism on Palestinian health share clear parallels with those of Indigenous populations in settings such as Australia and North America" (Tanous *et al.* 2023: 3). This is reflected in unequal access to healthcare "due to barriers such as the location of services (primarily located in Jewish Israeli towns), lack of public transportation, limitations in time and resources due to poverty, language barriers, and different access to education on preventive medicine" (Tanous *et al.* 2023: 7–8). Healthcare during conflict in Gaza is explored further in Chapter 6.

Older Arab Bedouin women living in southern Israel are a "doubly marginalized minority", as Shibli *et al.* (2021) put it: a minority within a minority (the Arab Muslim population). Living in both a geographical and social periphery they have poor access to healthcare because of transport difficulties and socio-cultural barriers. While there are community health centres, their opening hours are limited, as are staff numbers. As seen elsewhere in this book, mere location of a facility does not guarantee genuine access or utilization.

In a previous book (Gatrell 2023: 52–5) I sought to convey something of the inequitable treatment of Indigenous populations in the Global North, how this has deep roots in colonial history and is reflected in stark contrasts between these groups and white populations. Serious problems in accessing healthcare apply to Native Americans, to First Nations Canadians and to Aboriginal populations in Australia and Māori in New Zealand.

In the US the Indian Health Service (IHS)[32] exists to offer healthcare to Native Americans. Its mission is "to raise the physical, mental, social, and spiritual health of American Indians and Alaska Natives (AI/AN) to the highest level" and the stated vision is to ensure "healthy communities and quality healthcare systems through strong partnerships and culturally responsive practices". The gap between policy and experience, however, is rather wide. There is inadequate access to screening for breast cancer (mammography). There are structural barriers, including poor geographical accessibility to prenatal care and maternal health services, for example in the Northern Plains region (Montana, Nebraska, North Dakota, South Dakota and Wyoming), where there is a lack of culturally informed, women-centred care (Burns *et al.* 2023). Kroelinger *et al.* (2021) used GIS to explore the spatial accessibility to critical obstetric services in the US. Across the country only two-thirds of AI/AN women resided within 50 miles of these facilities, compared with almost 90 per cent of white women. This reflects the largely rural locations of AI/AN populations. Addressing the issue is far from straightforward, but the authors suggest that increasing incentives for healthcare professionals to practise in rural areas, getting state governments to help finance transport, and increasing the provision of telemedicine may all help.

More qualitative research sheds further light on problems of access for AI/AN populations. Reporters in the city of Sioux Falls, South Dakota, for example, conducted interviews and examined hospital records, finding that "patients would rather stay home

32. https://www.ihs.gov/

than risk getting care at Indian Health Service hospitals". Among several distressing stories is that from tribal health leader Spotted Elk, whose IHS doctor misdiagnosed the sore on his foot as a symptom of diabetes although it turned out to be bone cancer, likely resulting from exposure to toxic radiation at Fort McClellan Army base, Alabama. Both legs were amputated but the cancer returned to his collarbone and forearm. At the non-IHS hospital in Rapid City parts of the bone were removed and he was asked to return for follow-up visits. However, these were not covered by the IHS. "Fortunately, I didn't die of cancer in spite of IHS' lack of care", Spotted Elk said.[33]

The Canadian healthcare system was summarized earlier (pp. 41–2) but it is clear that First Nations people, whether living on reserves or in urban centres have poor access to healthcare services. Such access may be geographical; for example, Burnett *et al.* (2020) report on the challenges of journeys to health centres when roads are closed during winter months. Climate change is having an impact on ice roads on lakes in Northern Ontario, which are no longer freezing, restricting vital supplies of medicines to Indigenous communities. But journeys have other risks. In towns such as Thunder Bay, Ontario "it is not uncommon for Indigenous Peoples ... to experience violence while travelling to the city to access health care or education". There are other challenges, the authors reporting that some health professionals treat their patients with disrespect. "Compounded by racism and colonialism, many participants indicated that they had not developed long term and trusting relationships with health care providers" (Burnett *et al.* 2020: 5). In addition, some clinics showed a lack of flexibility over appointments. After a long bus trip with three small children one mother was required to reschedule after turning up 10 minutes late.

This links to the issue of decolonization (Gatrell 2023: 14–15), part of which requires involving members of First Nation communities in planning healthcare provision and acknowledging a role for traditional medicine (Eni *et al.* 2021). This is explored in considerable detail by Phillips-Beck and her colleagues (2020) who conducted almost 300 in-depth interviews with First Nations communities in the province of Manitoba. Findings include a long history of mistrust towards Canadian institutions, "navigating a system that devalues First Nation health and wellness", and "fundamental systemic racism" (p. 5) that is most clearly expressed by the stereotype that links First Nations identity to alcoholism. As one interviewee expressed:

> *They see your face and they assume that you are an alcoholic. My dad went up* [nearby town hospital] *and he had this woman doctor. And she's like, "I don't know why you come up here. This is not your heart, it's because you drink too much." My dad hasn't had a drink in, I don't know how many years.*
>
> (Phillips-Beck *et al.* 2020: 9)

33. https://eu.argusleader.com/story/news/2018/12/05/south-dakota-ihs-patients-share-medical-horror-stories-inadequate-care/1728836002/

For those travelling into the city (Winnipeg) it can be disorientating:

> *I was sent (to Winnipeg); by myself I go for whatever appointment I have then they're going to shove you out from there, to another section, drag you around ... What are you supposed to do? We're in a strange place I don't know my way around the city.* (Phillips-Beck *et al.* 2020: 13)

We thus see that "navigating" the healthcare system for Indigenous Canadians can create both geographical and socio-cultural disconnection (Horrill *et al.* 2018). For Eni *et al.* (2021: 2) "decolonization has a revolutionary potential that requires the dismantling of colonialism as the dominant model upon which Canadian society, and healthcare provision, more specifically, operate".

Māori populations in New Zealand have similar experiences. Systematic reviews of Māori healthcare (notably, Graham & Masters-Awatere 2020) suggest many failings, including not only overt racism and discrimination but a dismissive attitude to cultural and spiritual needs. Low-income participants in research studies listed financial costs, transport difficulties and practical problems such as arranging time off work or childcare: medical staff failed to appreciate the challenges of synchronizing employment and healthcare appointments. Even relatively 'minor' fees were a barrier to access, with low-income single mothers reporting having to choose between food and healthcare: "*That's half of our food for the week to go to a doctor and for me, it's not an option*". Travel times for rural dwellers were a significant barrier with one family who "*travelled over 100 kilometres ... then endured a long wait with some stressful behaviours needing to be managed*" (quotes taken from Graham & Masters-Awatere 2020: 197).

Dr Rachel Mackie, Chair of the Royal New Zealand College of General Practitioners Māori representative group says,

> We have known how the health system fails to deliver appropriate levels of care for Māori for decades, we constantly raise the issue, and it is still not being addressed. Equity is a major health concern and Māori are worse off because not enough is being done. The problem is not just in the hospitals either. The Ministry of Health's 2019/20 New Zealand Health Survey reported Māori adults had the highest prevalence of not being able to book an appointment at their usual general practice within 24 hours, which often will affect the whole *whānau* [the extended family group].[34]

34. https://www.rnzcgp.org.nz/news/media-releases/maori-tamariki-continue-to-suffer-most-from-health-inequities-new-research-shows/

In contrast, evidence suggests that Māori health providers offer practical and emotional support, including "displaying interest in the whānau and personal life" and exhibiting qualities such as "compassion, warmth, honesty, [and] respect, all of which had a positive impact on emotional wellbeing". Māori health providers were more affordable, assisted with practicalities such as transport and resulted in improved health outcomes. Aspects such as being able to "talk a little bit more freely", feeling understood, and having a connection with a Māori health professional who was "able to relate" were deeply appreciated" (quotes from Graham & Masters-Awatere 2020: 198).

Accessing healthcare for Australia's First Nations (also known as Aboriginal) women suggests that the same issues of remoteness and cultural insensitivity are at work as they are in the US, Canada and New Zealand. Research on maternity services (antenatal care) in Queensland between 2012 and 2015 (Fox *et al.* 2021) suggested that First Nations women were significantly less likely to attend for appointments or to receive psychological support if they had a mental health diagnosis. The authors conclude that "when it comes to Australian healthcare policy, First Nations women are not adequately supported. Rather, a long history of paternalistic government decisions have created barriers that actively inhibit engagement and attendance" (Fox *et al.* 2021: 2192). Requests to have access to traditional birthing practices tend to be ignored.

Gatwiri *et al.* (2021) put these issues in very sharp relief in telling the story of a 27-year-old pregnant woman from the Wiradjuri Nation who had made numerous visits to hospital but was dismissed as a likely drug addict. An inquest into her death confirmed that staff were racially biased. Indeed, the authors assert that "systemic and individual racism have been embedded within Australia's healthcare delivery since invasion in 1788" (Gatwiri *et al.* 2021: 2). The word "invasion" contrasts dramatically with conventional school textbook histories of the "discovery" of the continent by the "heroic" Captain Cook. One co-author of the cited paper says: "*Many of our people, don't feel safe in hospital. I've heard people say they would rather die than go to hospital where they are made sicker by encounters of racism*" (Gatwiri *et al.* 2021: 6).

Concluding remarks

This chapter has sought to offer a broad-brush picture of global healthcare expenditure and a description of the main types of healthcare system. Examples of the latter are examined further in the following two chapters where, first (Chapter 4), attention is given in particular to the UK and US. In both these countries this can only be an interim statement, since new governments (particularly the Trump presidency) can very quickly render such accounts obsolete. Nonetheless, the continuing "hit" being placed on the poorest members of society, via programmes of austerity (even if not named as such), remains a key part of the political economy of healthcare in these countries. The same feature applies to the growing reliance on private healthcare.

In Chapter 5 we see the same issues of inequitable healthcare, with detailed attention being given to five countries. Whether in the Global North or South there are particular challenges faced by Indigenous populations, and these have been outlined above. The colonial histories that have impacted on such populations have been highlighted in this chapter, as have attempts to repair these impacts via the decolonization of healthcare.

Particular populations, living in particular places at particular times, have seen their healthcare compromised, or at worst, denied, by the power exercised by some governments and interest groups. In large part, the latter applaud the marketization of such care, treating it as a commodity that only the market can address. Running through this chapter has been a thread of inequity. That thread continues to weave its way throughout the next two chapters.

Further reading

Chapter 7 ("Systems of Health Care") in Gatrell and Elliott (2015) covers some of the same ground as this chapter and has some useful background information on systems operating in both the Global North and the Global South. For an excellent comparison of 10 countries in the Global North see regular reports by the Commonwealth Fund.[35]

On the classification of healthcare systems Reibling *et al.* (2019) is worth consulting; they use multivariate cluster analysis to assign OECD countries to one of five types.

Christiansen (2017) offers a critical perspective on healthcare commodification and, in places, discusses Cuba's healthcare system. Privatization and its impacts are discussed in Turshen (1999: Chapter 3). Roderick and Pollock (2022) provide a succinct, but critical, account of recent developments in the NHS in England. See also the pressure group Patients 4 NHS website.[36]

For an excellent overview of issues of access to healthcare among Indigenous populations see Davy *et al.* (2016) but the more recent theoretical and empirical work described in this chapter should be consulted. The recent book by Sowemimo (2023) on racism and the need to decolonize healthcare is essential reading, while the National Collaborating Centre for Indigenous Health (NCCIH) in Canada has a superb paper on access to health services for Indigenous Canadians.[37]

35. Such as www.commonwealthfund.org/publications/fund-reports/2024/sep/mirror-mirror-2024
36. www.patients4nhs.org.uk/how-is-the-nhs-being-privatised
37. www.nccih.ca/docs/determinants/FS-AccessHealthServicesSDOH-2019-EN.pdf

4

GEOGRAPHIES OF ACCESS IN THE GLOBAL NORTH

> The development of technologies [has] worked hand in hand with the intensification of discourses of privatization ... whereby waiting as experience, as a source of meaning and as a form of care, became subsumed by the problems of too many waiting, and waiting too long. Bar-Haim *et al.* (2023: 7)

This chapter begins by examining varying levels of healthcare provision occurring in some countries in the Global North (Figure 4.1). In doing so it considers the distribution of the healthcare workforce in selected countries, with the main focus being the UK and US, and paying particular attention to the medical workforce and how some areas are "under-doctored" or classified as "underserved". The focus then shifts to the "consumer" and how, in an anti-collectivist context such as the US, some areas have relatively high proportions of their population who are uninsured.

Later in the chapter we examine issues of access in a collectivist context, with considerable attention given to the UK (and more specifically England) and how access to both primary care (in general practice and community dentistry) and secondary (hospital-based) care varies from place to place. The latter is illustrated with a particular focus on access to cancer care services. Despite that focus it is fair to say that issues such as waiting times apply to many other specialties.

Consequently, much of this chapter is about "waiting" (Bar-Haim *et al.* 2023). Invariably, one has to wait to see a family physician (general practitioner) for an appointment. You may not have to wait if admitted with a life-threatening condition to an emergency department (Accident & Emergency: A&E in a UK context) but if you turn up there unannounced there may well be a long wait to be seen and an even longer wait for a bed if you need to be admitted. If a primary care physician suggests you need to see a hospital consultant there may be a lengthy wait for such an appointment and a further wait if you need surgery. All these "waits" can vary according to place, and to social and economic circumstances. In a collectivist context, such as the UK, if you have money you can probably circumvent these waiting times by paying for private care (see pp. 81–2).

Waiting – whether for a consultation or for surgery – can be a very stressful time (Box 4.1).

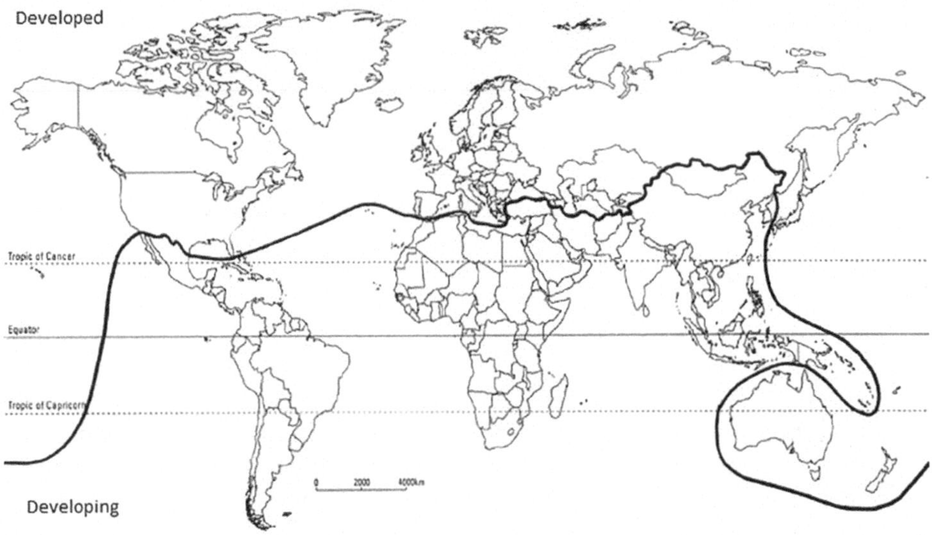

Figure 4.1 The "Brandt line", separating the Global North ("developed") from the Global South ("developing")
Source: Gatrell (2023: 5).

BOX 4.1 WAITING TO BE SEEN

While healthcare commissioners and governments collect and analyse data on waiting times there is a significant personal dimension to this, which only qualitative data can reveal. In Southwark, a London borough, people were asked about their experiences of waiting for hospital treatment (www.healthwatchsouthwark.org). Some were resigned to the need to wait but others were stressed because of the uncertainty of not knowing when they might be admitted. That caused stress in relationships and in mental as well as physical health. Others felt they were "fighting" the system. For example: "*If you want anything to happen you've got to push it yourself. But it's very difficult to push, because you don't know what to push, or where, or who to push ... It makes you very anxious also, because it goes on for a long time*" ... "*I just feel really awful ... and now I worry myself because they take long to provide me with information or they don't tell me what's happening properly ... I'm kind of scared of them now*". For others, having a supportive primary care physician helps: "*The only people that have really reached out, is my GP, because obviously they're fully aware of my condition ... GP has been very good, as well as the pharmacist. They've all been really good with me*".

Punton *et al.* (2022) illustrate how lengthy waits for mental health appointments have serious impacts on the health and well-being of young adults. As one of their student interviewees put it: "*It does put a strain on a lot of things to know that some medical conditions can be seen so quickly, whereas it almost seems as though mental health isn't classed as the same sort of severity as physical".* As the authors write: "waiting lists in mental healthcare are associated with a variety of negative consequences, including the development of maladaptive coping mechanisms and the emergence of negative or irrational beliefs" (Punton *et al.* 2022: 14).

Whether dealing with physical or mental health, family and friends can help, but alleviating lengthy waits for access needs organizational change.

Andrews and Evans (2008: 761) suggest that "medical geography's traditionally broad engagement with facilities and services ignores the workers who frequent and operate them". The following section seeks not to "ignore" the workers, although it does not address the "geographies in workplaces" that Andrews and Evans want to explore.

The unequal provision of doctors

A global picture of the healthcare workforce was presented earlier (pp. 36–7). Here, the focus is a national (mostly, in England) look at one category of the healthcare workforce (doctors), acknowledging that issues of supply concern other health professionals: nurses, pharmacists, dentists and allied health professionals. More specifically, the focus is on family physicians (general practitioners: GPs) who are often the first point of call unless an emergency arises.

In England there are well-known shortages of GPs, as confirmed in a report by the Nuffield Foundation.[1] Their analysis reveals that despite the (Conservative) government's target to increase the number of GPs by 6,000 between 2019 and 2024, between 2019 and 2023 there were actually fewer (848) GPs in England. There is a geography to supply in the UK (Figure 4.2), with practices in some regions (North West, Midlands, South East) having many more patients on their "list" (and therefore greater workloads) than elsewhere. For example, in 2022 north-east London had 2,057 patients per GP, compared with 1,342 in Devon in south-west England.

It is therefore of little surprise that the Nuffield Foundation speaks of a workforce "crisis" in the NHS. In 2014 the chair of the Royal College of General Practitioners in the UK asserted that: "The general practice [GP] workforce is unevenly spread across the country, with the fewest doctors in the most deprived areas, exacerbating health inequalities" (cited in Asaria *et al.* 2016).

What about other parts of the UK? The issue of access to GPs in Scotland is particularly acute in rural areas. Ian Kennedy, chair of the British Medical Association in Scotland

1. www.nuffieldtrust.org.uk/resource/the-nhs-workforce-in-numbers

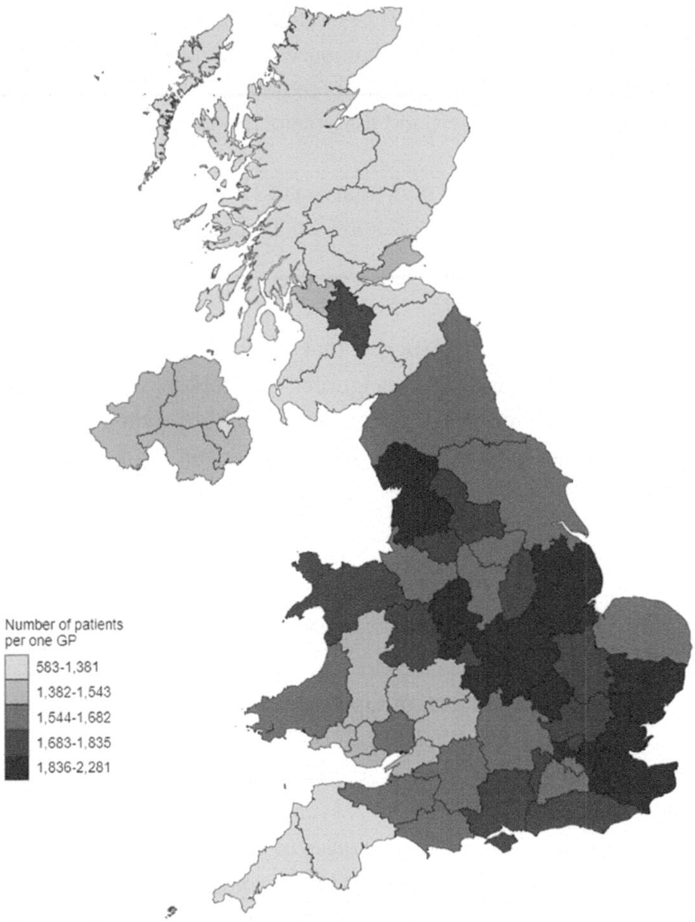

Figure 4.2 Number of patients per GP in the UK (2022)
Source: www.nuffieldtrust.org.uk/resource/the-nhs-workforce-in-numbers.

acknowledged there are "huge vacancies in Orkney, Shetland, Western Isles, Grampian, Highland, Borders … the rural–urban divide is getting greater".[2] Dr Kennedy himself works in the city of Inverness but he asserted "If I'm a rural GP, I am it. There isn't a local hospital nearby. If you are having a heart attack, it's a matter of me treating your heart attack. You are the doctor, you're the healthcare assistant, you're the nurse, you are the emergency service" (*The Guardian*, 3 January 2024).

GPs receive funding from the NHS, based mainly on the number of patients registered with them, although the formula that determines funding also takes into account other

2. https://www.theguardian.com/society/2024/jan/02/bma-scotland-chair-calls-for-urgent-action-to-address-shortfall-of-rural-gps

factors, such as the age of patients, "additional needs" (according to mortality rates) and rurality. However, this formula has been criticized for not taking sufficient account of the levels of deprivation in each practice area. The Health Foundation suggests that when the increased needs of patients in areas of high deprivation are allowed for, GP practices in more deprived areas of England are relatively underfunded (and under-staffed). In 2018/19 such practices received about 7 per cent less funding per patient than in those in less deprived areas.[3] There are growing workloads in areas of deprivation, for reasons of both demand (many of those living there have complex needs and multiple morbidities) and supply (difficulties in recruiting to areas of deprivation). In addition, there is evidence that areas with large numbers of ethnic minority populations have 37 GPs per 100,000 patients, about 15 per cent fewer than areas with low proportions of non-white populations (about 44 GPs per 100,000).[4] All these issues point again to the "inverse care law" referred to in Chapter 2. As Ashworth and colleagues (2021) put it, primary care funding "entrenches health inequalities".

At times, there have been financial inducements (one-off payments, occasional loans) to doctors to work in under-doctored areas. However, as Chekar *et al.* (2024: 742) point out, these do not "take into account the lived experience of working medical professionals, and while additional resource would be welcomed by many ... this alone is inadequate to resolve the problem".

There are factors other than national or regional funding that shape the geographical distribution of the healthcare workforce. Some of these relate to personal circumstances and choices about where to live, reflecting the "mental maps" or spatial preferences that individuals hold (Gould & White 1974). As with other professions, people want to feel welcome and safe in a new location and to develop a sense of belonging in a place that may encourage them to remain. Malatzky *et al.* (2020) stress the importance of this for workforce retention, particularly in the context of the rural healthcare workforce. However, Chekar *et al.* (2024) stress that there needs to be more flexibility for doctors in training to accommodate family circumstances, otherwise there are risks of trainees (particularly women) leaving the profession; such risks hardly enable greater workforce diversity.

Herrick (2023) writes in the context of the UK's NHS "Long Term Workforce Plan"[5] introduced by the Conservative government in 2023, that sought (among other things) to increase the healthcare workforce, while at the same time relying less on staff from overseas. The Plan is also concerned with the *nature* of the workforce, including replacing some primary care medical staff by less well qualified health professionals (so-called "Physician Associates"). This is proving controversial, as outlined in Welch (2024), whose

3. www.health.org.uk/publications/reports/doing-more-for-less
4. See www.theguardian.com/society/2024/feb/15/ethnic-minorities-in-england-have-worse-access-to-gps
5. www.england.nhs.uk/publication/nhs-long-term-workforce-plan/

book invites a close reading of the issues facing doctors working in the UK's NHS (see pp. 122–5 on the subject of Physician Associates).

What of the situation in the US? The US Health Resources and Services Administration (HRSA) designates as a Health Professional Shortage Area (HPSA) any geographical area, population group or healthcare facility that has a shortage of health professionals, whether these relate to primary care, dental care or mental health. There are almost 7,500 such areas in the US relating to primary care.[6] Many of these areas and facilities struggle to recruit, and retain, health professionals, creating underserved areas, not least in rural areas. Primary care HPSAs (pHPSAs) designations are based on four factors (Streeter *et al.* 2020): the ratio of population to providers; percentage of the population that is below the Federal Poverty Level; an infant health index (which includes data on the infant mortality rate and low birth weight rate); and travel time to the nearest healthcare centre. Such areas are associated with poorer health outcomes. Wang and Luo (2005) use the two-step floating catchment method outlined in Chapter 2 to identify underserved areas in Illinois but link measures of spatial accessibility to data on social disadvantage and healthcare needs.

Other countries are faced with similar issues of workforce distribution. Box 4.2 considers the example of France while Siegel *et al.* (2016) offer a description and analysis of service accessibility in Germany.

Does the provision/supply of doctors have any significant impact on health outcomes? Research in the US suggests that it may. Shi *et al.* (1999) analysed data for US states, finding a significant association between good supply of primary care physicians and lower mortality, greater life expectancy and improved birth outcome; however, their subsequent analysis at the level of 273 metropolitan areas (Shi & Starfield 2001) is less conclusive.

In Canada Lavergne and colleagues (2023) have traced equity in access to primary care (as evidenced by individuals' responses to the questions "do you have a regular medical care provider" and "do you have a regular place of care"?). They relate these yes/no responses to various predictors, including gender, social position, ethnicity, immigration status and self-reported health, and examine changes between 2008 and 2018. About 82 per cent of those on low incomes in 2008 said they had a regular medical provider, compared with 86 per cent on higher incomes, but while the latter percentage was unchanged in 2018 the percentage for those on lower incomes had declined to 79 per cent.

I say more about the movement of doctors in Chapter 7, but having discussed some issues relating to the *provision* of healthcare professionals, attention now turns to the impact this has on service *utilization*.

6. See www.kff.org/state-category/providers-service-use/health-professional-shortage-areas for a list and map of these by state.

BOX 4.2 MEDICAL "DESERTS" IN FRANCE

The experience of access to primary care in France mirrors closely that in England, with particular areas being underserved and people who are struggling to access a general practitioner visiting hospital emergency departments as an alternative. The French government defines a "medical desert" as an area in which fewer than 2.5 appointments per resident per year on average are offered. This reflects the declining number of GPs, falling from 97,000 in 2017 to an estimated 77,000 in 2025.[7] As in other countries there are inequalities. In 2013, the 10 per cent most well-off people had significantly better access to GPs than the 10 per cent least well-off.

The geography of this under-provision, and historical attempts to correct imbalances, is explored in detail by Chevillard and colleagues (2018). Financial inducements have been made to encourage GPs to work in underserved rural areas. Bonal and her colleagues (2024) widen the definition of primary care to include physiotherapists, nurses and pharmacies, with data collected for nearly 35,000 municipalities. They use the floating catchment method, with travel times estimated from municipalities to providers. Data on mortality and income were used to represent healthcare "need". Their detailed map that results from a cluster analysis (Bonal *et al.* 2024: 17) reveals areas that have both poor spatial accessibility but also high needs, particularly reflecting older populations. These areas are found mainly in parts of northern France, but are dispersed across the entire country. Better served areas are found in coastal regions and the larger towns and cities.

Accessing primary care: when can I see the doctor?

The Department of Health and Social Care in England funds local councils to set up branches of "Healthwatch", which seek to discover what communities want from their health and care services. In Blackburn, Lancashire, the local branch explored in 2023 the experiences of people living in the most deprived parts of the town. Various themes emerged from the focus groups and interviews. Most confirmed that it took under 15 minutes to get to their GP surgery but while "getting there" was not an issue, "getting through" – in terms of being able to have their call answered, or to make a suitable appointment – was, for three-quarters of respondents, much more problematic. Surgeries open at 8 am for bookings but as one person reported: "*Ringing up at 8 am just doesn't work for people – if you're working or taking kids to school, you're simply not free at that time*". An 86-year-old said: "*You can be up to number 46 in the queue so it's just easier to*

7. https://www.connexionfrance.com/news/frances-medical-deserts-pushing-more-gps-to-turn-away-new-patients/196228

physically go down to the practice to book one".[8] As a result, many people have given up on trying to get help from the GP and visit the local hospital A&E department as the default option. Others have sought alternative sources of advice and treatment. As the Blackburn report stated: "People wanted greater clarity about what accessible services are available and where, in order to stop their default option being Emergency Department because they know it is always open".

The issue of difficulties in getting access to (utilizing) primary care is a common theme throughout England, as elsewhere in the Global North, although what follows is largely about the situation in England. As noted above, waiting to get an appointment is one challenge, but on arrival at the clinic there are other challenges, such as: the time spent in the waiting room; the consultation time and the patient's satisfaction with that consultation; and whether the patient sees a different clinician every time they visit. All these issues are monitored in the annual GP–Patient Survey, undertaken by NHS England.[9] That survey contains a rich body of data for all GP practices in England and the online tool gives scope for comparing one practice with others, or with the national picture.

Among the many questions asked in the GP–Patient Survey are those concerned with seeking an appointment over the telephone. This is not straightforward. Nationally, the GP–Patient Survey suggested in 2024 that about half of those surveyed reported difficulties in having a telephone call answered. Clearly this varies from place to place. For example, my own practice in Lancaster (north-west England) suggests that 74 per cent of respondents had difficulties getting through, well above the national average. Contrast this with Dunster and Porlock in south-west England, where only 10 per cent of the population have difficulties getting through to a receptionist.

Many patients ask to see a particular healthcare professional from one visit to the next. Nationally, 40 per cent can do so. Again, comparing the same two practices, 25 per cent in Lancaster and 55 per cent in Dunster and Porlock seem able to have that potential continuity in care. This is due in part to practice size: the Lancaster practice currently has 41 GPs available, spread across several sites, compared with just five in Dunster and Porlock. But does continuity of care matter? Evidence from a recent study (Kajaria-Montag *et al.* 2024) that has analysed data from 10 million consultations in England, suggests that seeing the same GP improves patient health, reduces GP workloads and frees up appointments. It may also reduce the number of referrals to secondary (hospital) care. This finding is not restricted to England. Evidence from Norway (Jelin *et al.* 2024) confirms that, from the patient perspective, the key determinant of accessibility is seeing the same GP.

But what happens during the consultation? Is there any evidence that GPs spend less time with patients from poorer areas? Gopfert *et al.* (2021) have sought to answer this using a random sample of 1.2 million consultations in England between 2014 and 2016.

8. https://healthwatchblackburnwithdarwen.co.uk/wp-content/uploads/2023/07/Priority-Wards-Engagement-Report.pdf
9. https://gp-patient.co.uk/

They conclude that GPs in England spend less time with patients who live in deprived areas, regardless of their level of multimorbidity. The average consultation time was about 11 minutes and the difference between the least and most deprived areas was 0.5 minutes, but that has to be seen in the context of the very large dataset. The results lead the authors to conclude that "the inverse care law [Box 2.1] is alive and well in general practice in England" (Gopfert *et al.* 2021: e191).

There is evidence of an association between the proportion of ethnic minority populations and the proportion of all respondents reporting good overall satisfaction with GP services (Figure 4.3). This is an "ecological" study, however, based on areal units called clinical commissioning groups (CCGs) – now superseded by integrated care boards (ICBs) (pp. 39–41) – so it does not say anything about individual satisfaction. Nonetheless, "GP surgeries with the highest proportion of Asian/Pakistani respondents were the least likely to report good overall experience" (Magadi & Magadi 2022: 9).

I referred above to the stresses involved in waiting for an appointment. There are other waits involved in primary care, not least waiting to be called to see a doctor or nurse after arriving at the surgery. Kearns and colleagues (2020) refer to the waiting room as an "unexamined space". The layout and design (including artwork) can make such places less stressful for the patient, as can the staff (receptionists) working there if they show help, respect and consideration. Kearns *et al.*'s research in city practices in New Zealand reveals a range of experiences and emotions. For some, "bounded spaces (such as 'clinical' waiting

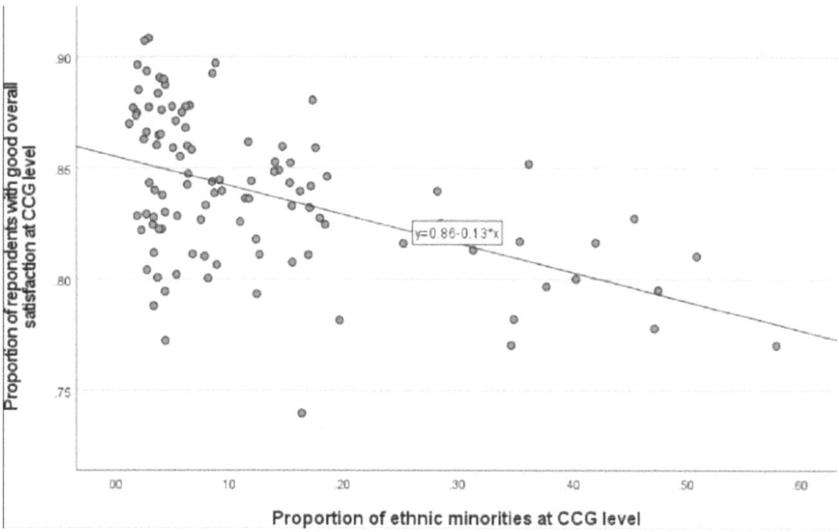

Figure 4.3 Overall satisfaction with GP services related to ethnic minority population in England (based on data for 2021)

Note: CCG: clinical commissioning groups.

Source: Magadi and Magadi (2022).

rooms and reception areas) are potentially problematic for people who experience social exclusion. Here, they can easily feel judged on the basis of appearance, financial 'means' and medical condition" (Kearns *et al.* 2020: 5). The authors call for waiting rooms to be more "permeable". By this they mean it should be possible to engage in activities while waiting to be called, allowing the individual to remain a person and not merely a patient. The more "sympathetic" waiting areas do of course provide reading matter (even if the magazines are over 12 months old!), toys for young children and music (even if not to everyone's taste).

As noted earlier (p. 63) the healthcare workforce comprises other professionals apart from doctors; healthcare can be accessed in other clinical settings, such as pharmacies. Aside from dispensing medications that a GP might have otherwise prescribed, these provide over-the-counter remedies but also vaccinations and professional advice. In England, the "Pharmacy First" scheme aims to have pharmacies carry out consultations and prescribe medications for selected conditions. The government website asserts that "Four in five people in England can reach a community pharmacy within a 20-minute walk and there are twice as many pharmacies in the most deprived communities, making access to care quicker and more convenient".[10] However, in England, out of a total of about 10,000 pharmacies, over a tenth of these have closed since 2007, putting additional pressure on GP services.[11] Further, the closures seem to have been occurring disproportionately in deprived areas. Between 2017 and 2023 the percentage reduction in pharmacies was about 11 per cent in the most deprived areas, but less than 6 per cent in the least deprived areas.

While pharmacies receive some core funding from the NHS this is not sufficient to cover costs. As one pharmacist in southern England put it: "It breaks my heart, because patients rely on us to provide a vital healthcare service, many of whom are elderly or vulnerable. However, we can't continue to carry on providing that service and care for our patients if this funding crisis is not addressed" (*The Guardian*, 29 March 2024).

Away from medicine, Box 4.3 examines access to another aspect of healthcare: dental care in the UK.

Accessing secondary care: how long must I wait?

It is impossible to review here the large literature on access to secondary (hospital) care so I focus attention on just one aspect – cancer care and treatment – and the determinants of access, before considering access to end-of-life (palliative care) services. It is important to note that those services do not cater solely for those living with cancer. A focus on the cancer pathway should not deflect attention from inequalities in waiting times for other conditions (Box 4.4). There are some online resources that can inform potential patients

10. https://healthmedia.blog.gov.uk/2024/02/01/pharmacy-first-what-you-need-to-know/
11. https://www.theguardian.com/politics/2024/mar/29/pharmacies-england-closed-poorer-areas-more-affected

BOX 4.3 ACCESSING A DENTIST: MORE THAN A FEW TEETHING PROBLEMS

In England, the NHS will (apparently) "provide any clinically necessary treatment needed to keep your mouth, teeth and gums healthy and free of pain". The NHS website goes on to suggest you can find "a dental surgery that's convenient for you" but adds the rider that you should "phone them to see if there are any NHS appointments available". Such a phone call is, however, unlikely to bear fruit. In late December 2023 over 83 per cent of dental surgeries in England were refusing to register new NHS patients and 71 per cent would not register those under 18 years of age. This lack of NHS provision is spatially patterned. In 2022, rural areas and areas of deprivation were least likely to have access to an NHS dentist. The City of Westminster in London has over six times the number of NHS dentists per head of population, compared with Ashfield in Nottinghamshire, the area with the lowest number in the country.[12]

Because of the difficulty getting an NHS appointment some patients have resorted to "DIY dentistry", pulling teeth out with pliers and using superglue on their gums. One disabled man "was in terrible pain and had been trying to get an appointment. He was managing his pain with paracetamol and gels. He was eventually offered an appointment ... but it was 60 miles away, and he couldn't attend because he is unable to travel far".[13] When a new NHS dental practice opened in Bristol in 2024 several hundred people queued round the block hoping to secure an appointment.

While there is no charge for consulting a GP or visiting emergency services, those accessing NHS dentists do have to make a financial contribution, according to the treatment required, which ranges from about £26 to over £300 (in February 2024) for more complex interventions. NHS dental care is free for children under 18, and for those under 19 and in full-time education, and also for pregnant women and new mothers. But this assumes dental practices are willing to accommodate these groups. In the absence of an NHS dentist locally, the options are to pay privately or do without treatment. There are significant geographic differences in the charges made by dentists. For example, root canal work can cost about £350 in Northern Ireland but over £750 in the east Midlands. Tooth extraction might cost £435 in eastern England but "only" £350 in the south-east and south-west.[14]

In February 2024, the then-UK government set up an initiative to pay 240 dentists up to £20,000 each as a "golden hello" to deliver NHS care in areas that are underserved. This was part of a plan "to make sure *everyone* who needs to see a dentist, particularly those who have been unable to access care in the past two years, will be able to do so, making

12. www.local.gov.uk/about/news/nhs-dental-deserts-persist-rural-and-deprived-communities-lga-analysis
13. https://www.theguardian.com/society/2023/oct/30/complaints-about-poor-nhs-dental-services-rise-66-in-five-years
14. https://www.theguardian.com/society/2024/dec/31/uk-patients-unable-to-get-dental-care-after-eye-watering-rise-in-private-fees

access to care faster and fairer"[15] (my emphasis). In addition, a new "dental vans service" was to be made available for selected rural and coastal communities that are presently underserved. However, by the end of the year the UK's National Audit Office reported that none of these had appeared and the "golden hellos" had attracted just one extra dentist. The Public Accounts Committee said these initiatives had been "a complete failure".[16]

Some researchers have used GIS to examine the spatial accessibility to dental practices. For example, Jo *et al.* (2021) report on public transport access to almost 9,000 practices in the UK but such "access" is of limited value if people cannot get an appointment provided by the NHS.

Clearly, in England – and, more widely, across the UK – there are more than a few teething problems in accessing dental care without incurring high costs.

BOX 4.4 WAITING FOR A NEW HIP

Hip replacement is a commonly used surgical intervention and can improve the quality of life for those suffering with severe joint pain.

In England there is a clear north–south divide in rates of hip replacement. Lenguerrand *et al.* (2023) examined where hip replacements (over 650,000) were undertaken between 2007 and 2017. They found that while the volume of activity had increased over 10 years, in the most deprived areas there were lower rates of surgery compared with the least deprived areas (Table 4.1).

The reasons for these inequalities are not always clear. Are they a function of differential provision in different areas, different referral patterns by GPs or different attitudes to the perceived benefits of surgery?

Waiting times for hip surgery tend to be longer for those with less education and on lower incomes. Waiting times vary from place to place. For example, in Wales those needing a hip replacement wait for about a year in many parts of the country, but almost two years in the Swansea region.[17] To deal with the demand a considerable number of operations are now outsourced by the NHS to the private sector; Kirkwood *et al.* (2024) report that between 1997 and 2019 about 15 per cent of hip replacements were undertaken in that way. The same authors report that the growing use of the private sector (see below, pp. 81–2) has increased levels of inequality. "The policy of outsourcing NHS care and expanding the number of private providers operates in favour of the rich to the detriment of the poor" (Kirkwood *et al.* 2024: 6); those needing a hip replacement and living

15. https://healthmedia.blog.gov.uk/2024/02/07/dental-recovery-plan-everything-you-need-to-know/
16. https://www.theguardian.com/society/2025/apr/04/plan-increase-access-nhs-dentists-england-complete-failure-mps
17. www.bbc.co.uk/news/uk-wales-65265684

Table 4.1 Rates (per 10,000) of hip replacement in England

IMD quintile	*2007*	*2017*
Q1 Most deprived	18.7	23.9
Q2	24.9	30.4
Q3	29.1	37.8
Q4	30.6	40.8
Q5 Least deprived	31.2	42.6

Note: IMD is the Index of Multiple Deprivation.
Source: Lenguerrand *et al.* (2023).

in a deprived area were more likely to be treated in an NHS hospital rather than a private hospital. However, this study looks at *areas* of deprivation, not personal circumstances and it remains to be seen whether an individual is much exercised about where they are treated or what impact any treatment centre has on subsequent quality of life.

The same issues arise when looking for a knee replacement and, again, it depends where in Europe you live. Lengthy waiting times in England reflect "decades of under-investment in NHS staff, beds and equipment, which is leaving it trailing behind other European countries. For knee replacements, the median waiting time in England is 142 days. In Italy, it is fewer than 50 days".[18]

In the US a study on individuals with federal health insurance showed that Black patients were 30 per cent less likely to undergo hip replacement surgery than white patients, after standardizing for age and gender (Ryan-Ndegwa *et al.* 2021).

---

of likely waiting times. In England, the NHS website has a facility to search, by area and hospital, the average waiting times for first appointments and treatment for selected specialties, although information is variable and depends on whether hospitals choose to supply that information.[19]

Cancer diagnosis and treatment varies internationally in advanced economies. Comparisons of the UK, Australia, Norway and Canada reveal that, between 2012 and 2017, patients in the UK waited longer for treatment than in other countries. Moreover, this varied within the UK. There was a shorter average waiting time for chemotherapy in England (48 days) compared with Scotland (65 days), while the waiting time to begin radiotherapy was 53 days in Northern Ireland but 81 days in Wales.[20] There is marked spatial variation among ICBs – of which there are 42 in England (see above, pp. 39–41) – in whether cancer treatment targets are met. One such target is that 85 per cent

18. https://www.theguardian.com/society/2024/nov/27/bone-on-bone-agony-the-cruel-reality-of-facing-a-three-year-waiting-list-for-a-new-knee
19. www.myplannedcare.nhs.uk/
20. https://www.ucl.ac.uk/news/2024/feb/uk-cancer-treatment-falls-behind-other-countries

of those diagnosed with cancer should begin treatment within 62 days (two months) of an urgent referral. In 2023 no ICB met this target. Some areas, including Surrey and Kent in south-east England, reached up to 77 per cent but others, particularly in the Midlands (Lincolnshire, Shropshire, Leicestershire) managed only 50 per cent.[21] The reasons for these delays are many and varied, ranging from "behavioural" explanations (delays in seeking treatment, for example) to "structural" determinants (variations in service provision). In terms of the latter, shortage of staff and beds or "health provider-initiated delay" seems to be a key factor, certainly in the UK.[22]

Although over 20 years old, a study in south-east England (Robinson *et al.* 2005) revealed striking differences in waiting times for radiotherapy across different treatment centres. Examining data for over 600,000 cancer cases between 1992 and 2001 the proportion of those waiting 60 days for treatment ranged from 44 to 71 per cent, although this varied according to the type (site) of cancer. Further, the waiting times increased during that 10 year period.

But there are delays earlier in the cancer pathway. For cervical cancer screening there are gender-based disparities in England, with a so-called "postcode lottery". In London, only 61 per cent of eligible women had been screened, compared with 73 per cent in the north-east of England.[23] There appear to be disparities in terms of the intention to attend for such screening, as a study in the UK suggested (Wilding *et al.* 2022). Younger women, white women and those living in less deprived areas were more likely to report their intentions to attend for screening, while previous attendance was also inversely related to area of deprivation.

Some studies have compared levels of screening for cervical cancer among non-immigrant and immigrant populations. A good example comes from Finland (Idehen *et al.* 2018) where, between 2010 and 2012, about 94 per cent of Finnish women had been screened, compared with 79 per cent among Russian-born women and 64 and 41 per cent respectively for Kurdish and Somali immigrants. While letters inviting women (including immigrants) for screening are sent to all women aged 25–65 years the rates are clearly very different. The authors suggest these variations are in part due to language proficiency, with Russian women having a better understanding of the Finnish language. Somali and Kurdish women may be less familiar with such screening if it has been unaffordable in their countries of origin.

In the US Castellano and her colleagues (2022) provide a useful online tool for exploring geographic variation (by metropolitan statistical area) in screening for cervical cancer (and other data relating to cervical cancer).[24] This reveals interesting inter-state

21. See the map produced by Pfizer: www.pfizer.co.uk/files/Cancer-waiting-times-heatmap-Oct-2023.pdf
22. https://news.cancerresearchuk.org/shorthand_story/cancer-waiting-times-who-are-the-long-waiters/
23. www.theguardian.com/society/2024/apr/22/almost-600000-in-england-awaiting-gynaecological-treatment-figures-show
24. See: https://geo-analyzer.org/#/dashboard

differences; for example, in South Carolina screening rates for women aged 18–44 years are over 60 per cent while in neighbouring North Carolina the rates are under 50 per cent. Elsewhere in the US Agénor and colleagues (2024) suggest we cannot ignore social inequities, and in particular structural racism as a determinant of variations in screening for cervical cancer (Box 4.5).

Yet geography – the location of patients relative to treatment centres – cannot be ignored. If cancer centres are increasingly centralized (see above, pp. 49–50) then inevitably people have to travel longer distances for treatment. Those with the means to bear the costs may well be willing to trade those costs against the possible benefits from accessing more specialist care in larger cancer centres. Obrochta *et al.* (2022), in a study of Californian cancer patients, labelled this the "travel time paradox". However, they also reveal that 15 minute increases in journey time are associated with a 24 per cent increase in the risk of under-treatment for Black patients, relative to white patients, and a 35 per cent increased risk of delayed treatment for those living in the poorest neighbourhoods

---

BOX 4.5 STRUCTURAL RACISM AND CANCER CARE

Statistical evidence concerning the relatively poor access affecting people of colour with cancer must be complemented by hearing directly from individuals. Suha Ahmed, aged 35, arrived in Northern Ireland from Sudan in 2021. She said that, after struggling to get an appointment with her GP and visiting the local A&E hospital department, she was eventually diagnosed with cancer and since the diagnosis was late it had spread. In her words: "*Accessing health care was the first difficult thing I faced in this country. I rang my doctor almost every day to see him face-to-face but I couldn't get through or get an appointment*". She continued: "*I would say please, please – especially to the doctors – please, if you have a patient, don't look at the colour or where he is from – just look to his symptoms, because if you lose time it is so hard*".[25]

Sowemimo (2023) writes at length about the impact of racism on healthcare. Recall from the discussion of access in Chapter 2 that one dimension was "acceptability", or the perception of services. Sowemimo notes that 60 per cent of Black British people consider that their health is not as well protected by the NHS, compared with white people; this varies by gender, with 78 per cent of Black women having that belief. She suggests that the same is true in the US, where there is fear and suspicion of white doctors, as well as differences in the prescribing of pain relief among Black and white patients (Sowemimo 2023: 87). Elsewhere, she writes that "women's pain, and especially Black women's pain, is being silenced" (95), particularly for those giving birth (103).

---

25. https://www.bbc.co.uk/news/articles/cq5xnv0zlqgo

relative to those in wealthier areas. As the authors note, in the US healthcare system (above, pp. 44–9) patients' healthcare utilization is shaped by insurance status and the choices that better-off people can exercise.

Longer travel times can affect outcomes for cancer patients. A Scottish study suggests that those who have to travel further for care – rural and island dwellers – are more likely to die within the first year of diagnosis. Better contact with services is required, which may only be possible through improved digital healthcare (see pp. 157–61 below). Yet it is not only rural populations who incur disadvantages. In the US, urban populations on low incomes or without health insurance or affected by structural racism have difficulties accessing cancer care and are more likely to experience worse outcomes despite services being geographically proximate. "Structural determinants for cancer care delivery (e.g., access to income, transportation, childcare, and health insurance) become especially nuanced in densely populated areas like New Jersey where the geographic availability of oncology specialty providers is high" (McGee-Avila *et al.* 2023: 153). As noted in Chapter 2, simply having services close by is no guarantee of "access".

Accessing palliative care

Palliative care is the provision of support and care to people who are dying and their families. While it embraces those with other conditions, much of the literature on access to palliative care services focuses on those with cancer. Such care can be offered at home or in hospital but hospices are a valued setting – in which case it is of interest to learn about access to such services and in particular whether such access is inequitable.

As with other aspects of cancer care there is plenty of evidence that geographical proximity plays its part in accessing services. A study in England and Wales (Gatrell & Wood 2012) mapped small areas where the supply of hospices (in terms of bed numbers) that look after adults was below average and potential demand (in terms of cancer deaths) was above average. These were then related to data on relative deprivation. Results revealed that although urban areas are relatively well served, large parts of (rural, coastal) England have relatively poor *potential* access to hospices, and their needs may be unmet. Chukwusa *et al.* (2020) developed these ideas further, using individual rather than aggregate data, for England as a whole. Drive times from patients' usual place of residence to the nearest hospice and hospital were estimated and these were used as explanatory variables to model the individuals' place of death (whether hospice, home or hospital). The findings support the rural "gap" in hospice access identified by Gatrell and Wood (2012). Patients in both rural and urban areas who lived more than 10 minutes' drive from a hospice were less likely to die in such a setting, compared to those who lived within 10 minutes (Figure 4.4). One way of dealing with this inequality is to use hospice-at-home services or telehealthcare (see Chapter 7), which can improve access to palliative care in more rural areas.

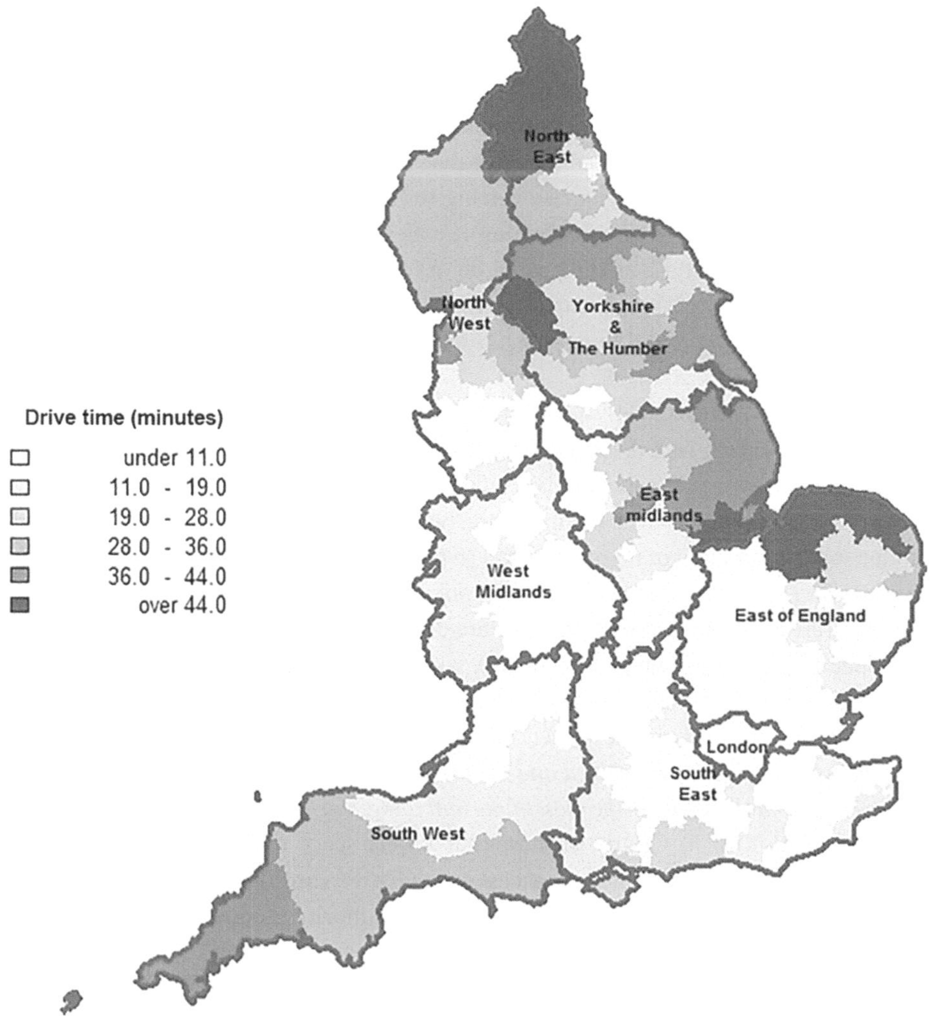

Figure 4.4 Drive times to nearest adult in-patient hospice in England in 2014 (darker shading refers to longer drive times)
Source: Chukwusa *et al.* (2020), licensed under Creative Commons.

In the US, Carlson and colleagues (2010) undertook a nationwide study of geographic access to hospices, based on estimated drive times between census tracts and hospice locations. Almost all areas were within one hour's drive time from at least one hospice but this varied according to census characteristics. Areas with higher proportions of well-educated people and on higher incomes, but also with higher proportions of Black people, were all within 30 minutes' drive time from a hospice. Inevitably, the more rural states (such as Montana, Wyoming, and North and South Dakota) revealed poorer geographic accessibility, with more than a third of their populations living at least 30 minutes from the nearest hospice. But this study relates very much to provision, not service use.

Distance is not only geographical; there is an emotional distance or separation between the person who is dying and their family members. In rural areas such as parts of British Columbia it is not only measured distance that proves a barrier to accessing palliative care; road conditions in winter make driving to hospices (or hospice carers travelling to patients' homes) extremely challenging (Castleden *et al.* 2010). In addition, not all hospices are as welcoming as they could be. As one of the respondents in the British Columbia study put it: "*I'm not satisfied with the rooms at all. The care* [and] *the nurses are fine, but it's pretty awful to be going to such a barren room and those are your last days*" (Castleden *et al.* 2010: 287).

Bayley and Crowther (2024) seek to study the emotional geographies of hospice care, noting that there may be a deep affection for such places ("topophilia") but for some the opposite feeling of dread ("topophobia"), reflecting the physical location of the hospice and the care some provide. Some patients see the hospice as "*more like home than a hospital*" but for some it is a place of no return: "*You go there you are not coming back. I've seen the hospice. That's how I understood it. No coming back out*" (Bayley & Crowther 2024: 3). Yet their research confirms that hospices are deeply embedded in local communities as "therapeutic landscapes" (above, pp. 9–10), with strong affection for the care they provide. In similar vein, Moore and colleagues (2013) have explored, using photo-elicitation interviews, the sense of place experienced by day care patients in an English hospice. As one man puts it: "*I feel very relaxed and I enjoy coming here, it's pleasant, it's relaxing and you feel safe. And that to me is the most important thing. You feel like you're amongst friends*" (in Moore *et al.* 2013: 5). Clearly, the hospice is a social space, as much as a physical place.

A systematic review of unequal access to palliative care services across the globe suggested that very old people, those from ethnic minority groups, and those living in rural and socio-economically deprived areas are under-represented (Tobin *et al.* 2022). Indigenous populations in Australia and New Zealand, for instance, are less likely than white populations to receive hospice care. Here, and elsewhere, the relations between hospices and those who refer patients to them (hospital doctors, general practitioners) are key in determining access. As French and colleagues (2023: 516) put it: "Hospice and other specialist palliative care organizations could look to foster closer integration with hospitals, as well as community settings, as a way of initially connecting with patients in more socially deprived areas".

Accessing emergency care

Inevitably, because hospitals dealing with those suffering from trauma (for example, resulting from serious accidents) are few and far between there is a geography to accessing such services. Among many studies Lilley and colleagues (2019) have modelled geographical access to emergency care in New Zealand. Using GIS, they assess the differential access (according to age, population density, ethnicity and deprivation) of population sub-groups living in small areas. Their results suggest that 16 per cent of the New Zealand population (about 700,000 people) lack timely access to advanced-level hospital care, either by road or via helicopter. This access is particularly acute for Māori and older New Zealanders, along with those living in the South Island. There is a clear gradient with deprivation: almost three-quarters of those living in the least deprived small areas are within 60 minutes of an emergency centre that deals with advanced trauma compared with just over half of those in the most deprived areas. Of course, as the authors note, such services are located to serve densely populated areas, where demand is likely to be higher and a well-equipped and skilful workforce exists. Nonetheless, "the unequal distribution of healthcare resources across New Zealand provides a further pathway for health disparities for Māori and rural populations: difficulties in achieved access to healthcare for these sub-groups are already well documented" (Lilley *et al.* 2019: 6). Studies elsewhere confirm that rural populations have relatively poor access to trauma centres. Carr and colleagues (2017) suggest that, in 2010, almost 30 million Americans lacked access to a major trauma centre (using a 60-minute threshold) and that areas with higher concentrations of vulnerable populations (including those uninsured, on low incomes and in rural areas) were disproportionately affected.

Many hospitals in England make it clear that attending A&E is not appropriate for minor issues (Figure 4.5). But for some people the A&E department appears a reasonable

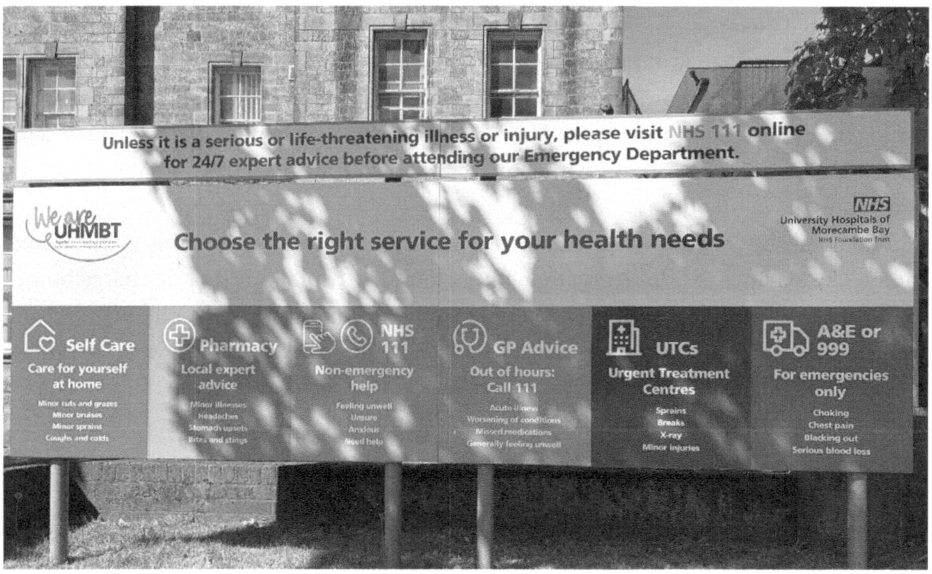
Unless it is a serious or life-threatening illness or injury, please visit NHS 111 online
for 24/7 expert advice before attending our Emergency Department.
We are UHMBT
Choose the right service for your health needs
NHS
University Hospitals of Morecambe Bay
NHS Foundation Trust
Self Care
Care for yourself at home
Minor cuts and grazes
Minor bruises
Minor sprains
Coughs and colds
Pharmacy
Local expert advice
Minor illnesses
Headaches
Stomach upsets
Bites and stings
NHS 111
Non-emergency help
Feeling unwell
Unsure
Anxious
Need help
GP Advice
Out of hours: Call 111
Acute illness
Worsening of conditions
Missed medications
Generally feeling unwell
UTCs
Urgent Treatment Centres
Sprains
Breaks
X-ray
Minor injuries
A&E or 999
For emergencies only
Choking
Chest pain
Blacking out
Serious blood loss

Figure 4.5 "Choose the right service for your health needs" (Royal Lancaster Infirmary)
Source: Author's photograph.

action if obtaining a primary care appointment proves very challenging (as discussed above) or if the hospital is closer than the primary care provider.

In England emergency calls are categorized according to whether the situation is life-threatening or less serious; in the former case (including, for example, a cardiac arrest or respiratory failure) the target mean response time is 7 minutes and 90 per cent of the time an ambulance is expected to arrive within 15 minutes. Inevitably, there is a geography to this, as a BBC News report revealed in 2019.[26] Across Britain as a whole the average response time for rural areas was 11 minutes 13 seconds, compared with 7 minutes 14 seconds in urban areas. Such differences are critical for patients with a heart attack but the growing number of defibrillators being located in rural settings can help – providing people are trained to use them. In the UK the iconic, disused red telephone boxes are a popular location.

Analysing almost 600,000 emergency calls it appears that rural, coastal locations have lengthy response times. The longest response time was for Wells-on-Sea in north Norfolk. "One former community responder in Wells told the BBC he resigned because of the length of time he was left with badly-injured patients before ambulance crews arrived".[27] Press stories report regularly on lengthy waits. For example, *The Guardian* newspaper recounted the 10-hour wait for an ambulance in Wales to arrive at the home of 76-year-old Dave Strachan. When an ambulance did reach him and get him to hospital it was too late. At the inquest the coroner said: "The time it took for an ambulance to be dispatched and arrive and convey him to hospital meant that there was a missed opportunity to have probable life-saving medical treatment." This is not a rare event. In 2022 over 500 patients (people in accidents, with heart attacks) in England died after a delayed ambulance response.[28]

As with Wendy's story in the introductory chapter, waiting for an ambulance to arrive is only one aspect of the patient "journey" to hospital. What do we know about the waiting times once the ambulance delivers the patient to the hospital? And for those who present themselves to A&E departments how long do they have to wait, and are there inequalities in waiting times?

In the English NHS the standard is that 95 per cent of people attending A&E should wait no more than four hours for either admission to a hospital ward or discharge home. Performance against this target has been declining for many years and the most recent data from the King's Fund suggested that, in 2023–24, only 58 per cent of attendances were seen within four hours. The pressures are worse in winter months. In December 2023 and January 2024 over 98,000 patients waited more than 12 hours for a bed to

26. https://www.bbc.co.uk/news/health-47362797
27. Ibid.
28. www.theguardian.com/society/2024/nov/13/nine-hours-52-minutes-did-dave-strachan-ambulance-wait-cost-him-his-life

become available after the decision to admit – and this after already waiting to be seen on arrival at A&E.[29]

Using data for 2016–17 Turner *et al.* (2022) explore inequality in waiting times in major English emergency departments, finding that patients from the most deprived areas wait longer than others and are less likely to be admitted to a hospital bed, although some choose to leave without treatment. The reasons for this are varied, and include individual, patient-level factors (some people communicate their needs better). However, results "are consistent with physicians systematically assigning lower clinical priority to more income-deprived patients compared to less deprived patients with equivalent objective healthcare needs … Our results may point to unconscious bias by physicians driving inequalities, rather than patient-physician communication problems". Crucially, "our results suggest that the NHS principle of 'equal access for equal need' is not being upheld in English Emergency Departments" (all quotes from Turner *et al.* 2022: 15). Such inequity is not restricted to England. Research in Swedish emergency departments found that low-income patients arriving and reporting chest pain were more likely to be assessed later than those on higher incomes (Herlitz *et al.* 2023).

Hospital "provision" does not merely mean getting an appointment and being seen. It also means having access to a safe environment, which includes buildings being safe. The BBC has reported on "thousands of potentially harmful incidents [in 2023] including critically-ill patients being moved when rainfall came through the ceiling". Such incidents also include sewage leaks, floods and failing equipment. "Imperial College Healthcare NHS Trust in London had the largest high-risk repair backlog in 2022–23 at more than £392m. A high-risk repair 'must be urgently addressed to prevent catastrophic failure or major disruption to clinical services', according to NHS Providers".[30]

The privatization of cancer care

As noted earlier, in order to access secondary healthcare in the UK some people will "go private", using either their own savings or using private healthcare insurance that they have purchased. This reflects an unwillingness to incur potentially lengthy waiting times for treatment. In England, NHS targets for cancer treatment are consistently being missed. There are many stories of those opting, usually unwillingly, for private healthcare. For example, Alan Gregory was told that the waiting list for prostate surgery was 18 months but he waited only two months for surgery after a private consultation,

29. www.bbc.co.uk/news/health-68306477/
30. https://www.bbc.co.uk/news/uk-england-68214879, 21 February 2024.

at a cost of £8,000. "I resent being put in a position by Tory failures to have to pay", he said, adding that he was aware that he was fortunate to be able to afford it.[31]

The Private Healthcare Information Network reports that between 2018 and 2023 almost 300,000 people used private healthcare insurance to pay for chemotherapy treatments, with almost 14,000 using their own funds to pay for it. The companies that provide private healthcare insurance have, inevitably, been keen to fill the gaps that have arisen because of lengthy waiting lists. The insurance company Aviva recorded a 58 per cent increase in sales of health insurance premiums in January–July 2023, netting income of £86 million. The company's chief executive gleefully announced that she saw "literally opportunities everywhere".[32]

The privatization of cancer care is even more extreme in the US. Perry and Bernasek (2024: 3) argue that profits are made from "expensive cancer treatments not from the prevention of cancer or the search for a cure"; the latter is "not part of the capitalist healthcare industry's approach to cancer care". Their empirical analysis at the state level uses various measures of corporate capitalism for hospitals and the health insurance and pharmaceutical industries. Relating these measures to data on cancer mortality reveals significant positive associations; their results do not imply causation, but they are highly suggestive. More generally, Booth *et al.* (2023) suggest that, too often, commercial interests, rather than those of patients, are a key driver of cancer research and care. Worryingly, a "substantial proportion of industry revenue is used for marketing campaigns to influence patients, policy makers, and oncologists, irrespective of clinical need" (Booth *et al.* 2023: 833).

Concluding remarks

A focus on cancer has meant that the considerable literature on access for many other conditions has been overlooked, although I referred above (pp. 39–40) to some of the unevenness in access to assisted reproductive technologies (fertility treatment). Missing from this chapter is anything on access to care for people living with dementia, or those with mental health issues. On the latter, evidence in England suggests that there are clear geographical inequalities, with some mental health patients being sent on distant placements, far from their homes and families.[33]

31. https://www.theguardian.com/society/2024/mar/08/my-gp-suggested-it-britons-explain-why-they-went-private-for-surgery
32. https://www.theguardian.com/business/2023/aug/16/big-opportunities-in-expanding-private-health-cover-amid-nhs-strain-says-aviva-boss
33. https://www.theguardian.com/society/2024/nov/21/mental-health-patients-harmed-by-being-sent-to-units-far-from-home-report-finds

Equally, there is interesting research being done on access to organ transplantation. Evidence from the US suggests that patients awaiting a liver transplant and who live in higher income neighbourhoods and have private health insurance are much more likely to receive a transplant, while poorer patients in rural areas are less likely to have had an assessment for transplant suitability (Yilma *et al.* 2023).

What this chapter has revealed, however, is unequal – and in some cases inequitable – access to healthcare, whether that be primary, secondary or emergency services. Such variation in access occurs despite the availability of universal healthcare in most countries of the Global North.

Further reading

The geographer Danny Dorling has written extensively on inequality, including unequal health and healthcare, particularly in a British context. See, for example, Dorling (2023: 163–88). Although now somewhat outdated Baggott (2004) has a fine overview of healthcare in Britain and is well worth reading. More recent is Exworthy *et al.* (2023).

Very useful independent sources on healthcare in the UK are provided by the Kings Fund and the Nuffield Foundation, while for the US the Kaiser Foundation is another valuable, independent source on health policy.[34]

On the discourses of "waiting" (oriented towards the UK's NHS but of wider relevance) I strongly recommend Bar-Haim *et al.* (2023).

The term "postcode lottery" referred to on p. 39 is quite widely used to denote local and regional inequalities in service provision. Redhead and Lynch (2024) have an excellent piece on the history of its use. Curiously, equivalent terms such as "zipcode lottery" do not appear to have entered the geographical lexicon.

For an important recent paper on the various barriers to accessing cancer services in western Canada see Horrill *et al.* (2025).

Sítima *et al.* (2024) have a recent overview of the literature on the equity of access to palliative care services, although their search criteria limited it to only 14 studies.

34. www.kingsfund.org.uk, www.nuffieldfoundation.org/?s=healthcare and www.kf.org

5

GEOGRAPHIES OF ACCESS IN THE GLOBAL SOUTH

> Private medical care is exclusively clinical, and it lacks meaningful connection to public health and the social measures needed to improve the health of the majority.
>
> Turshen (1999: 42)

I referred in Chapter 2 to the so-called "inverse care law" that describes the relationship between healthcare need and the lack of resources allocated to those people – and those places – most in need. As we shall see in this chapter this relationship applies as much to those living in the Global South as it does to those living in the Global North. There are demonstrable inequities in the matching of supply and demand of skilled healthcare workers in the Global South. Countries in sub-Saharan Africa have one-quarter of the burden of global disease but only 3 per cent of the world's skilled healthcare workers (Kasper & Bajunirwe 2012). The same authors note that 32 of these countries do not have the World Health Organization (WHO) recommended minimum of 23 skilled healthcare workers for every 10,000 population.

In a previous book (Gatrell 2023: 66–70) I wrote briefly about this mismatch, and referred to specific case studies. In particular, I discussed the work of Moosa and colleagues (2014), who interviewed health professionals trained in various African countries but who preferred employment in Europe or South Africa. The reasons they gave for leaving included poor working environments, shortages of equipment and probable poor career progression. The consequences of these perceptions for the provision of primary care in particular are severe. In Chapter 7 I discuss further the factors that lead to the migration of health professionals from the Global South to the Global North.

In this chapter I first ask about the attempts to move towards universal health coverage (UHC), a stated target of the Sustainable Development Goals. It is stating the obvious, but health is a key component of development. Brief attention is given to the relative roles of so-called "vertical" and "horizontal" programmes of healthcare, before exploring in more detail issues of access to healthcare in five countries: Brazil, China, India, Mozambique and the Democratic Republic of the Congo. This selection mirrors that in

Gatrell (2023: Chapter 2) which considered the spatial patterning of health inequalities in the same countries. Here, the focus is less on inequalities in ill-health; rather, on inequitable access to the care that might help alleviate poor health.

Universal health coverage?

The WHO defines UHC as meaning "that all people have access to the full range of quality health services they need, when and where they need them, without financial hardship".[1] Among the 17 Sustainable Development Goals (SDGs) Target 3.8 is to "achieve universal health coverage, including financial risk protection, access to quality essential health-care services and access to safe, effective, quality and affordable essential medicines and vaccines for all";[2] see also Gatrell 2023: 22–4 for a brief introduction to the SDGs. To support these aims a large group of countries, global health organizations, non-governmental organizations (NGOs) and philanthropic organizations have come together to form UHC2030 whose mission is "to accelerate sustainable progress towards universal health coverage (UHC), focusing on building equitable and resilient health systems that leave no one behind and that provide the foundation to achieve health security".[3]

The relationship between UHC and other SDG goals is shown in Figure 5.1. Crucially, the graphic stresses how important it is for health systems to be "strengthened" (robust and resilient). In particular, and of relevance to this chapter, UHC can contribute to equity in health outcomes (SDG 3).

The definition of UHC given above presents a laudable goal, but one that is as unachievable in the Global North as in the Global South; we saw plenty of evidence in the previous chapter to support this assertion. But what evidence is there to suggest that countries are at least on track to attain universal healthcare coverage? The WHO offers a sobering picture:

> The world is off track to make significant progress towards universal health coverage ... by 2030. Improvements to health services coverage have stagnated since 2015, and the proportion of the population that faced catastrophic levels of out-of-pocket health spending increased continuously since 2000. This global pattern is consistent across all regions and the majority of countries.[4]

1. www.who.int/health-topics/universal-health-coverage
2. https://sdgs.un.org/goals
3. www.uhc2030.org/who-we-are/about-us/
4. www.who.int/news-room/fact-sheets/detail/universal-health-coverage-(uhc)

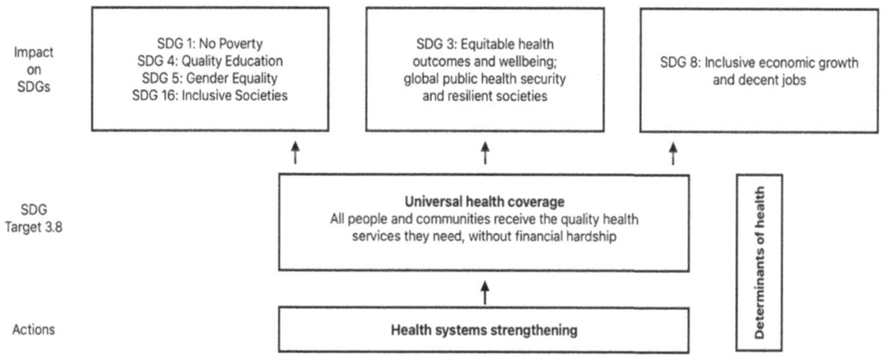

Figure 5.1 Relationship between universal health coverage and SDGs
Source: Based on Kieny *et al.* (2017).

As suggested in Chapter 2, structural adjustment policies have hardly helped to improve coverage. To make such improvements, according to the WHO, requires a focus on primary healthcare; put differently, it requires a focus on horizontal, as opposed to vertical, programmes (Box 5.1).

The "death of distance"?

Before turning our attention to case studies I think it is important, in a geographical text, to attend to the role that geographic access still plays in many parts of the Global South.

In an influential book, the economist Frances Cairncross (1997) wrote that new communication technologies have led to the "death of distance"; she argued that such technologies have "obliterated" geographic distance as a significant determinant of how we conduct business and social interactions. While we examine such technologies in Chapter 8 it is important to recognize that, for many in the Global South, distance is still a constraint on how healthcare is accessed. From the many examples in the literature consider just three; these focus on access to maternity services, clearly crucial since their provision and use can determine infant (and maternal) health outcomes.

First, Tanou and colleagues (2021) explore the provision and utilization of antenatal care in Benin, West Africa. Using both health survey data and GIS the authors look at the distance (straight-line, by road and estimated travel time) between the places of residence of women who had given birth in the past five years, and the nearest health centre. Outcome variables included number of visits to an antenatal clinic and whether the woman gave birth at such a facility. After controlling for potential confounding factors

BOX 5.1 HORIZONTAL AND VERTICAL HEALTHCARE

Put simply, "vertical" healthcare means a focus on providing care and treatment for specific diseases and conditions, such as HIV or malaria, while "horizontal" programmes are more concerned with the provision of wider-ranging, generic healthcare, with attention given to primary healthcare and improvements in health determinants (such as clean water and sanitation). As Turshen (1999) has noted, until the mid-1980s most countries in Africa followed the Alma Ata proposals (above, p. 50) to focus on primary healthcare, but from the late 1980s the neoliberal agenda saw a contraction of the public sector and support for selective vertical programmes. Turshen writes that such strategies "do not share the objectives of primary health care to deal with power, ownership, equity and dignity" (Turshen 1999: 44) and documents the failure of such strategies in several parts of the Global South.

Turshen traces a declining role for the WHO in the mid-1980s and how its role in health policy was overtaken by the World Bank. The latter, she argues, took an instrumental view of health and healthcare, stressing the benefits to the economy rather than social welfare and promoting vertical rather than horizontal programmes. Writing over 25 years ago she says: "With the initiative in international health passing from public health specialists to bankers and financial underwriters, national health policy is increasingly set and monitored at the international level" (Turshen 1999: 132). However, in its written documents at least, the World Bank is perhaps changing its tune, suggesting in 2024 that it "supports countries efforts to achieve universal health coverage through stronger primary health systems and provide quality, affordable health services to everyone – regardless of their ability to pay".[5]

NGOs have been criticized for giving too much attention to vertical programmes and insufficient attention to improvements in basic infrastructure and developing workforce capacity.

there were significant associations between use of maternity services and the distance measures.

Second, qualitative research in Malawi (Nyando *et al.* 2023) explores a range of factors affecting the perceived likelihood of pregnant women (during the first trimester) attending for antenatal care. While difficulties arranging visits, lack of partner support and negative previous experiences of healthcare workers were perceived as barriers, so too were travel distances. As one 28-year-old woman said: "*We started antenatal* [care] *late because some of us stay far from the hospital and transport was a problem, it's more than seven km, we do not have money, we are poor*" (Nyando *et al.* 2023: 9). But, as we

5. https://www.worldbank.org/en/topic/universalhealthcoverage

have seen elsewhere, getting to a health clinic does not necessarily mean the women will be seen promptly. A 26-year-old said: "*We also get tired because we report at the facility around 6 am but health workers assist us very late. They start work around 10 am, which discourages us from starting ANC early*" (Nyando *et al.* 2023: 10).

Third, the same issues arise in a study conducted in Somaliland (in the Horn of Africa, yet to be formally recognized as a country). Abdiwali and colleagues (2024) interviewed healthcare providers as well as pregnant women, in and around the largest city, Hargeisa. The main barriers that emerged from interviews were a lack of awareness about antenatal care facilities, a lack of social support from partners and cultural beliefs. But distance from facilities and lack of transport figured too. A 30-year-old woman says:

> *This is my first visit to ANC service; my place is far from here. I need to have my usual checkup, which is very important for my health and my baby's health. However, it is difficult for me to find transportation easily. I prefer to do a checkup when I come around for other purposes, like going to the market.*
>
> (Abdiwali *et al.* 2024: 7)

History matters

We cannot understand the structures of healthcare in many countries of the Global South without knowing something of the history of colonization. In a colonial healthcare system there are two populations (settler and colonized), with the former given priority. Typically, this led to better-resourced hospital-based healthcare for the colonizing population and under-resourced provision for those being colonized, whose own expertise and approaches to healthcare saw little acknowledgement.

Healthcare in colonial Africa favoured urban areas where European populations had settled, leading to a neglect of rural areas. Such unevenness has continued in the postcolonial era where, as Farmer (2020) has discussed at length, control of the spread of disease (rather than healthcare) has been the norm ever since the "scramble for Africa" began in the later nineteenth century. He writes, "there was little in the way of post-primary education or medical care in occupied West Africa" (Farmer 2020: 252), with most care, certainly in rural areas, relegated to missionaries. In Nigeria such "settler preference" created a notable disparity between urban and rural areas in terms of healthcare provision, a gap that persists. Other writers offer a similar account:

> The health systems resulting from decolonization processes are characterized by limited access to care, the strong presence of an informal sector and a public system generally centred on hospitals. They have a structural presence of international NGOs compensating for the shortcomings of a largely underfunded

system. Colonial care systems imported Western methods, rejecting the benefits of local practices and know-how.[6]

The same issues have characterized the South African healthcare system. During apartheid the minority white population secured better access to healthcare than the majority Black population living in "homelands" "that detached the poorest areas from regions with better healthcare infrastructure" (Stuckler *et al.* 2011: 165). Post-apartheid the country inherited a healthcare system that was wholly inequitable, and despite government policy since 1999 the inequalities between the richer and poorer parts of the country have been maintained. "We found that South Africa's distribution of health spending was consistent with the inverse care law observed in other poor countries, according to which regions with greater health needs receive fewer health resources" (Stuckler *et al.* 2011: 170).

In some of the case studies considered below we highlight workforce issues. Sriram and colleagues (2021) discuss how the policies for regulating the healthcare workforce in India are rooted in the colonial period. The ways in which the British regulated medical training before independence in 1947 have affected relations between doctors and Indigenous practitioners, as well as relations between the federal government and states. Traditional practitioners of medicine in India were displaced by an imposed colonial model of Western medicine. Sriram *et al.* (2021: 7) argue that "even today, medical education struggles to shake off the metropolitan, urban orientation of curriculum and is failing to make graduating physicians more attuned to the needs and requirements of the local communities and primary health centres". Box 5.2 seeks to clarify briefly what is meant by "traditional healthcare", and examples appear later in the chapter when particular countries are considered.

Recent history matters more

As suggested above, it is important to take a long view of the geography of healthcare in the Global South, with particular attention to its colonial underpinnings. Of equal importance is to consider the ways in which access to healthcare is now being undermined by the abandonment of support from the US under the Trump administration. One of President Trump's initiatives has been to withdraw US funding for the World Health Organization.

Before Trump gained power the US donated more to global health than any other country, totalling about US$12 billion a year; yet this is only 0.1 per cent of the federal budget. The funding was directed via several departments, mainly the US State

6. www.altersummit.eu/analyse/article/commodification-of-health-the-challenge-facing-health-systems

BOX 5.2 TRADITIONAL HEALTHCARE IN THE GLOBAL SOUTH

The World Health Organization defines traditional healthcare (and medicine) as "the sum total of the knowledge, skill and practices based on the theories, beliefs and experiences indigenous to different cultures, whether explicable or not, used in the maintenance of health as well as in the prevention, diagnosis, improvement or treatment of physical and mental illness" (WHO 2019). Separate, but related, we can define complementary or "alternative" care as practices that are not part of biomedical care, some of which (acupuncture, for example) are commonly used in the Global North (see Brown *et al.* 2018: 82–5). The WHO report cited above has detailed country reports on the use of traditional care. Note that, in the above definition, there is a clause "whether explicable or not", suggesting that there remains scepticism as to the efficacy of traditional treatments. Regardless, an equity argument (and certainly a decolonizing perspective) suggests that traditional care should be acknowledged as a component of overall care. Patwardhan and colleagues (2023: 1) note that integrating traditional care into conventional healthcare systems "has the potential to promote universal wellbeing, affordability, *access, and equity* in line with the principles of planetary health" (my emphasis).

A good introduction to the geography of traditional healthcare is provided in Phillips (1990: ch. 4), although this is inevitably somewhat dated. A classic paper by Good (1977) introduced the study of traditional medicine to health geographers, noting that in many countries of the Global South "modern" medicine formed "a rather small and unimportant element of the total available health care" (Good 1977: 705).

Department and the Agency for International Development (USAID). Some resources went direct to countries (major recipients were Nigeria, Tanzania, Mozambique, South Africa, Uganda and Zambia) others to multilateral agencies such as the WHO and United Nations. Some funding was for specific diseases such as HIV/AIDS (through PEPFAR, the President's Emergency Plan for AIDS Relief), malaria and maternal and child health. Of the $12 billion funding in 2024, 44 per cent was for HIV/AIDS but 11 per cent was assigned to maternal and child health where the stated aim is to "mitigate maternal, newborn, and under-five deaths" and to "strengthen integration of maternal health services with family planning and *improve equity of access to and use of services by vulnerable populations*" (emphasis added).[7]

The US provided about 42 per cent of the overall global funding for international health assistance in 2023, followed by the UK (12 per cent), Germany (8 per cent) and Japan (7 per cent). As indicated in Box 5.3, funding for maternal and child health is under significant threat.

7. www.kff.org/global-health-policy/issue-brief/10-things-to-know-about-u-s-funding-for-global-health/

BOX 5.3 THE GLOBAL GAG RULE

In 1984 the US Republican administration under President Reagan introduced a policy to ban global health funding given to NGOs if they intended to use such funds for abortion-related healthcare, even when the funding might also be used for contraceptive services, HIV prevention and maternal health. Formally called the "Mexico City Policy" it has become known as the "Global Gag Rule" (GGR) (as it inhibits or "gags" NGOs from campaigning on such policies). The International Planned Parenthood Federation (IPPF) has been a key opponent of the GGR stating it "will never support policies which actively restrict or violate an individual's right to bodily autonomy, including the right to safe abortion".

Although the GGR was rescinded under President Biden, on 24 January 2025 President Trump reinstated it, ensuring also that it cuts a wide range of funding for global health. Writing before Trump's re-election Lane *et al.* (2021: 1805) said:

> The integrated nature of healthcare, particularly in low- and middle-income settings, makes it difficult to target one specific area without unintended consequences. Existing literature on the policy suggests broadly negative impacts on the health of those in affected countries, with long-term detrimental effects to social and economic infrastructure.

In a wide-ranging review Mavodza *et al.* (2019) document numerous examples of the impacts of the GGR on, for example, HIV/AIDS and child and maternal health. They conclude that "the GGR is dismantling health systems by causing confusion about its practical implementation; unraveling integrated systems; diminishing qualified staff and crucial resources; silencing necessary advocacy voices and spaces; and reducing health service provision – including but not limited to family planning services" (Mavodza *et al.* 2019: 19).

Lane and colleagues (2021) suggest that the GGR reflects a neo-colonial perspective on women's health and healthcare in the Global South.

We now turn to consider the geography of access to healthcare in five countries.

Brazil

Brazil is a federal republic that comprises 27 states, grouped into five macro-regions (Figure 5.2), and is a middle-income country with a population of 214.3 million in 2021. A public healthcare system, SUS (Sistema Único de Saúde: "United Health System") was introduced in 1988, providing free healthcare funded through taxation. This certainly led to improvements in a range of health indicators, such as infant mortality, across all

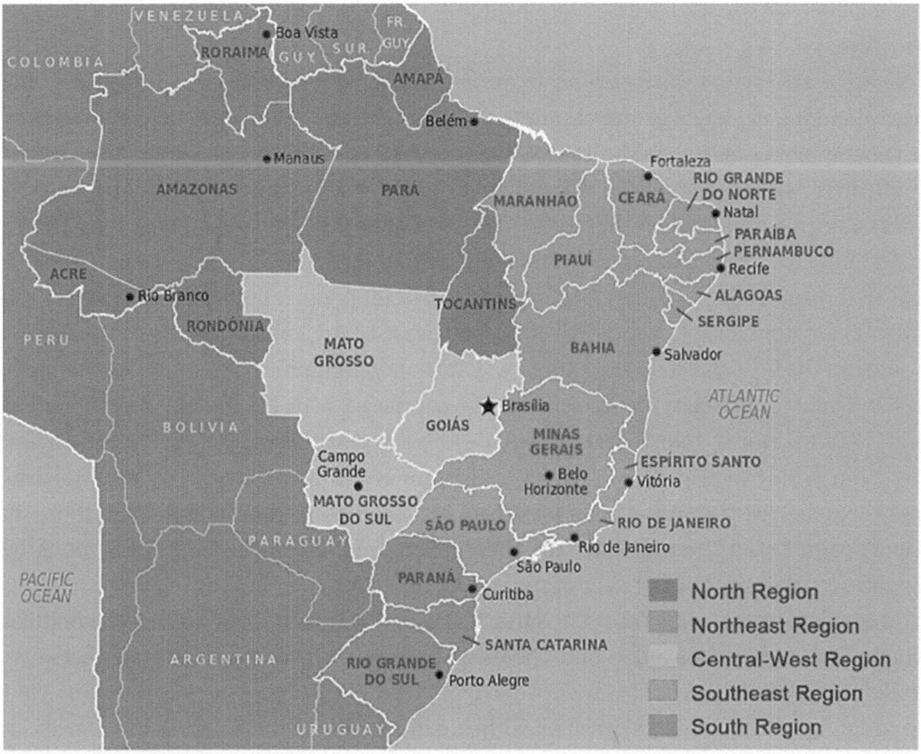

Figure 5.2 Brazil: regions and states
Source: Gatrell (2023: 30).

regions (Castro *et al.* 2019). Between 2016 and 2022 the country was led by conservative governments, with Presidents Michel Temer and Jair Bolsonaro, the latter displaced by the more moderate Luiz da Silva in 2023 who has revitalized the Family Health Strategy (a flagship of the SUS) that Temer and Bolsonaro had previously cut in order to encourage privatization and impose austerity. The historical evolution of the SUS between 1988 and 2019 is described by Castro *et al.* (2019) but also by Machado and Silva (2019) who have decried the policies of the right-wing governments.

The SUS was established on the basis of a need to provide universal and equal access to healthcare. It also proposed the decentralization of primary healthcare to the 27 states, and further, to 5,565 municipalities. A key component was the Family Health Strategy (FHS) that has provided primary care in these areas and in small neighbourhoods. Ortega and Pele (2023) describe the FHS as the largest community-based primary healthcare programme in the world, serving about 60 per cent of the population (over 130 million people). They also outlined the threats that the SUS (and its flagship FHS) faced from the neoliberal reforms discussed in Chapter 3, which saw an enhanced role for the private sector.

Despite the stated aim of SUS to promote equality of access to healthcare, the overwhelming evidence in Brazil points to consistent and enduring regional inequality in geographic access to healthcare (whether provision or utilization), with a clear north–south divide. These inequalities mirror income inequalities in the country. Martins (2024) offers a degree of optimism that the overall level of healthcare inequality in the country is declining, albeit slowly. Nonetheless, he points to inequality in the provision of medical staff. In 2014 there were 19.4 doctors per 10,000 people, but this varied across the five main regions, as follows: North 10.3, Northeast 13.0, Central-West 19.6, South 22.1, Southeast 34.4. At the state level there was further geographical variation; for example, in São Paulo (Southeast) the figure was 25.7 compared with 8.4 in Pará (North region) and 7.8 in Maranhão (Northeast region). de Oliveira and colleagues (2017) confirm that the main problems with the Brazilian healthcare system are the scarcity of physicians and the poor distribution of such professionals. They point out that, in 2014, those 39 municipalities having more than half a million people (and comprising 29 per cent of the population) had over 60 per cent of the country's doctors.

These data mirror those on basic infrastructure; while only 3 per cent of the population in São Paulo state lived in households without access to the general water network, in Rondônia (North region) it was over 51 per cent. This unevenness is the same with regard to the distribution of private healthcare insurance. In the Southeast region about 35 per cent of the population had such insurance, compared with 13 per cent in the North (data from 2013).

Salles and colleagues (2023) have undertaken to compile a detailed, and up-to-date picture (updated monthly!) of the provision of healthcare in Brazil. It includes geographically disaggregated data on the workforce and nature of facilities and infrastructure. Such data are publicly available and provide a rich source for quantitative geographical analysis. Alves and colleagues (2023) provide similar data, specifically for primary care.

Amaral *et al.* (2017) map in detail the provision of healthcare equipment in 2010, including machines for dialysis and magnetic resonance imaging (MRI), but also hospital beds. They estimate the distance between each municipality and the nearest facility providing particular equipment or beds and consider the balance between supply and demand for each state. Table 5.1 shows the percentage of municipalities within each major region without beds or dialysis machines, assuming a maximum distance travelled of 50 km. Clearly, the North is relatively lacking in access to hospital beds and dialysis machines; the paper maps the distribution across all municipalities, and the geographical disparities are clearly revealed at that scale.

In what follows we first consider in more detail access to primary care, then secondary (including emergency) care, before paying particular attention to the access offered to Indigenous populations in Amazonas and other states.

Table 5.1 Percentage of municipalities in Brazil in 2010 without hospital facility coverage (beds and dialysis machines) within 50 km

Region	*Beds*	*Dialysis machines*
North	20.0	82.6
Northeast	12.8	63.9
Centre-West	7.7	74.9
Southeast	17.3	27.8
South	5.0	28.2
Brazil	12.6	47.9

Source: Amaral *et al.* (2017: 11).

In order to improve the quality of care available to service users some governments have introduced performance incentives. Kovacs and colleagues (2021) consider whether payments made to providers, as part of Brazil's National Programme for Improving Primary Care Access and Quality (PMAQ), have improved or worsened healthcare disparities. A PMAQ score (based on indicators including patient satisfaction and level of antenatal care) was calculated for each of almost 14,000 primary care teams. Before bonus payments were awarded to these teams, those in the more disadvantaged Northern region had lower scores than those in the South and Southeast. While there was a positive association between the quality scores and average income in the areas they covered, these differences narrowed between 2011 and 2019. It appears that "pay-for-performance" incentives helped because they explicitly rewarded teams working in poorer areas.

In cities such as São Paulo the organization of the FHS is based on clearly defined catchment areas, with patients assigned to a healthcare facility within a specific territory (Iosti 2020). But this appears to be very much an administrative convenience, with little recognition of prior healthcare use or of the difficulties prospective patients have in negotiating hilly topography or accessing adequate public transport. Those living close to another catchment dislike the fact they cannot access a closer facility. As one resident complained: "*Why has it changed? Because the one here ... is much closer ... this post [facility] is very far away for us!* [...] *My God, it's much further away*" (Iosti 2020: 5).

Lopes *et al.* (2016) consider access to treatment for depression, suggesting that almost 80 per cent of those diagnosed with depression receive no treatments such as psychotherapy or antidepressant medications. Again, this is spatially patterned, with 90 per cent of those with depression living in the North left untreated, compared with 68 per cent in the South. Access to appropriate drugs in the public health systems was higher in the South (55 per cent) than the North (35 per cent). The same disparities exist for expert provision, there being 1 psychiatrist for every 15,000 people in the South, yet only 1 per 80,000 in the North. But there were other inequities: "despite the higher prevalence of depression among non-white skinned individuals, we found that being white increased the likelihood of receiving any treatment for depression" (Lopes *et al.* 2016: 7).

Exploring patterns of healthcare utilization from two survey dates (2013 and 2019) Szwarcwald and her colleagues (2021) find that regional inequalities are evident, with the highest use (such as a medical visit within the last two weeks) in the Southeast and South and the lowest in the North (and having controlled for income). As others have pointed out, this inequality reflects an unequal distribution of healthcare resources; there are unmet needs in the poorer regions. For example, de Andrade *et al.* (2022: 16) suggest that rates of preterm births are higher in those municipalities where there are staff shortages:

> The ability of health professionals to offer care is more strongly linked to reported pre-term birth levels than is the regional distribution of equipment or supplies. These results emphasize the importance of ensuring the presence of sufficient clinical staff and human resources, especially in the most resource-limited areas of the country.

Both Peroni *et al.* (2019) and Nogueira *et al.* (2019) have explored geographical variation in SUS screening for breast cancer (mammography). The former show that relatively wealthy states (such as São Paolo and Santa Catarina) have over 94 per cent of women aged 50–69 screened, while poorer states in the north (Amapa and Pará) have fewer than 15 per cent screened. This is partly because the wealthier states and regions have more hospitals and oncologists providing cancer care and treatment. Brazil has nearly 1.5 cancer hospitals and 23 oncologists per million people but these vary by region, with 7 oncologists per million people in the North to 32 per million in the Southeast. The same inequalities apply to infrastructure, including the distribution of mammography equipment, MRI equipment and CT scanners. In a devastating conclusion they write that "patients' right to health is systematically violated at different stages of the patient pathway" (Peroni *et al.* 2019: 11).

In a related paper Nogueira *et al.* (2019) have mapped, for 438 "micro-regions" (groups of municipalities), the percentage of mammograms for women aged 50–69 years (Figure 5.3). Clearly, the regional picture painted above masks considerable spatial heterogeneity. Interestingly, the authors point to an association with income inequality: a 1 per cent increase in the Gini index is associated with a 0.6 per cent reduction in mammography in a given micro-region; in other words, the greater the level of inequality in a micro-region, the lower the utilization of mammography.

But there are other factors limiting patients' cancer journeys. Treatments including radiotherapy and chemotherapy require frequent hospital visits and long distances may be involved, costing both money and time off work or caring responsibilities.

Large parts of Brazil, including the Central-West and North regions, and rural parts of the Northeast, do not have access to cardiac diagnostics (such as stress ECG and catheterization), despite there being quite high rates of mortality from acute heart disease

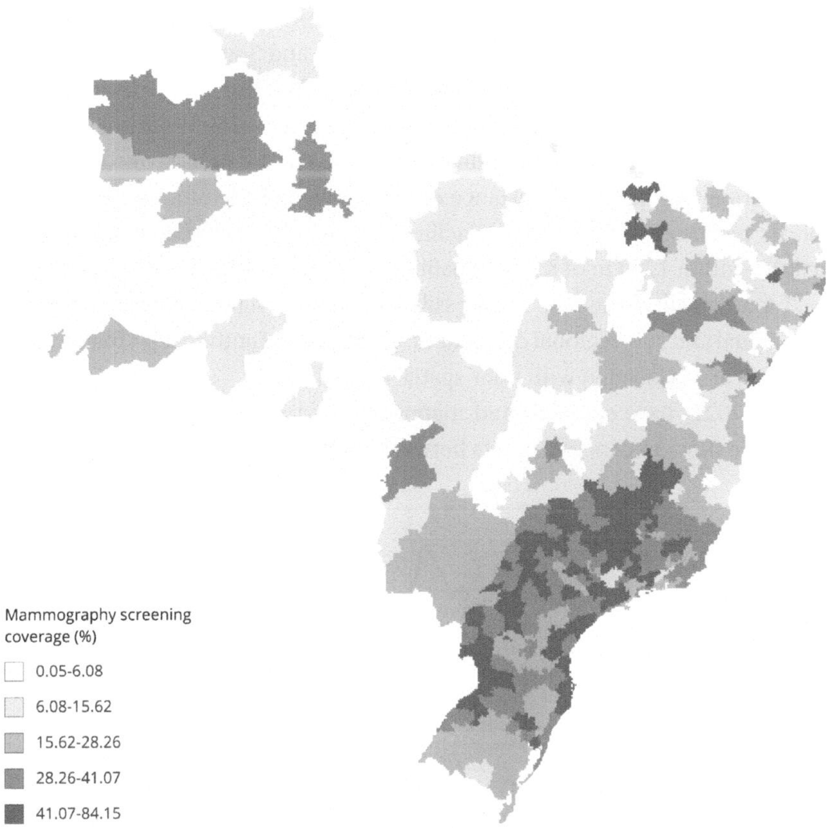

Figure 5.3 Distribution of mammographic screening coverage among women aged 50–69 years in 2010–11 by health micro-region (n = 438), Brazil
Source: Nogueira *et al.* (2019: 7).

(Hertz *et al.* 2019). Even in regions with good access (South and Southeast), the centres undertaking testing are clustered in the large cities, with those living more than two hours away having poor access. Clearly, if those with heart disease are poorly diagnosed there will be elevated mortality rates. There needs to be an expansion of testing taking place in hospitals located in poorly served areas. Hertz *et al.* (2019: 13) conclude: "As Brazil faces rising rates of risk factors for coronary artery disease that accompany rapid development, optimizing use of resources for cardiovascular care will become only more important".

Vissoci *et al.* (2019) have looked at spatial variation in the provision of surgical care for children. They note a clear disparity in the paediatric surgical workforce, with no more than 0.26 paediatric surgeons per 100,000 children in the poorer North and Northeast but up to 0.68 per 100,000 children in the wealthier South and Southeast regions. Such regional variation is independent of socio-economic status. The authors use the two-step floating catchment area (2SFCA) method referred to above (pp. 18–19) to map spatial accessibility. A radius of 120 km surrounding each care facility is used to define the paediatric population within a travel distance of two hours and the number of hospital beds available for paediatric surgery at each facility is calculated. The capacity ratios of all available facilities within 120 km of a municipality are summed to create an accessibility index for each municipality. The map of accessibility to first-level hospitals (Figure 5.4) reveals clear regional and sub-regional differences. Crucially, the authors find that under-five mortality rates are associated with poor spatial accessibility.

Fonseca *et al.* (2021) have explored and mapped – for two time periods (2009–10 and 2017–18) – the flows of cancer patients between municipalities (places of residence

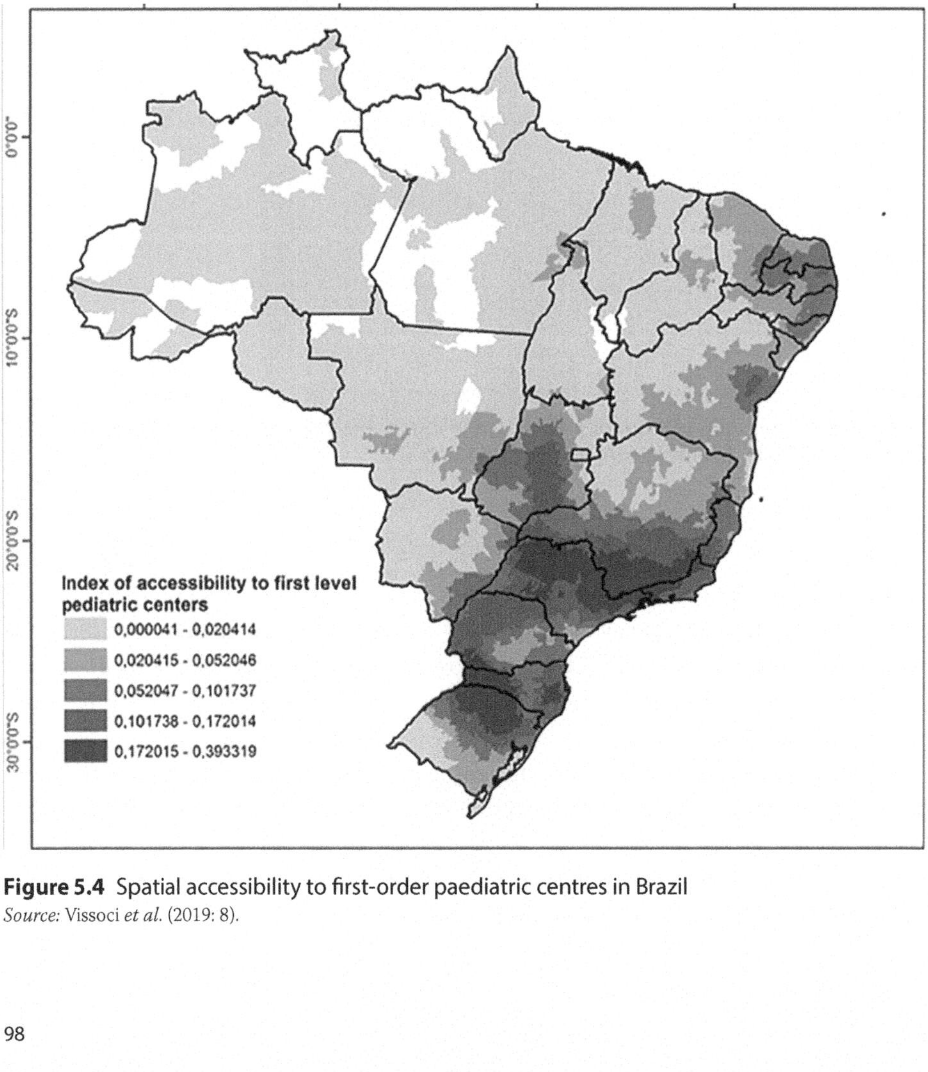

Figure 5.4 Spatial accessibility to first-order paediatric centres in Brazil
Source: Vissoci *et al.* (2019: 8).

and locations of hospitals that provide chemotherapy, radiotherapy or surgery). In both time periods over half of all patients had to travel outside the municipality in which they lived; on average, distances travelled, regardless of cancer intervention, were on average about 165 km, but 1 per cent travelled over 1,000 km. Those patients living in the North region travelled the furthest, while for those in Amazonas state the distances travelled for radiotherapy and chemotherapy increased over time. Inevitably, given the concentration of facilities and expertise in major urban centres, and the fact that Brazil is a "country with continental dimensions" (Fonseca *et al.* 2021: 13), people will have to travel far to access care. Establishing cancer centres in places of need, notably in the North, would help alleviate regional disparities.

Several writers have examined access to emergency care. Rocha and colleagues (2017) looked at both paediatric and adult intensive care units (ICUs), as well as access to emergency obstetric services. Nationally, more than 14 and 30 million people lived more than 120 km from centres that had an ICU or paediatric ICU, respectively. Paediatric ICUs are concentrated largely in São Paulo, Rio de Janeiro, the south of Minas Gerais and Parana, while large areas in the North, Northeast and Central-West regions are left unserved. Access to emergency obstetric care was better, with over 80 per cent of the total population living less than 60 minutes from such centres. In general, what the authors find is serious spatial disequilibrium, with wealthier regions well served by both large and small hospitals. They suggest that such "overlap" is wasteful of resources that could be deployed to overcome such geographical inequality.

Turning to Indigenous healthcare, Gomes and colleagues (2024) have undertaken qualitative research on Quilombola communities in the north of Minas Gerais state; the Quilombola are descendants of African-Brazilian enslaved people. There are almost 400 communities, dispersed among over 155 municipalities in the state. The authors undertook interviews in six communities and these revealed the importance of popular knowledge in healthcare, knowledge of herbs and other plants that has been transmitted down through generations. As one woman put it: "*We usually make home remedies. My backyard is like a pharmacy, there's a remedy for everything, my neighbors ask for them and I give them some*" (in Gomes *et al.* 2024: 4). Accessing more formal biomedical care is constrained by transport difficulties. As a male respondent said: "*it's very far from the city (São João da Ponte). The roads are in very bad condition, full of potholes, and during the rainy season, it's impossible to pass. We suffer a lot when we need medical attention*" (Gomes *et al.* 2024: 7).

These findings are echoed by Rodrigues and her colleagues (2021) in a study set in a remote rural community in the most western state, Acre. These authors caution that it is often the historical and cultural background of Indigenous populations that shapes healthcare, not simply whether more formal services are accessible. Nonetheless, transport difficulties certainly constrain access; as one interviewee put it: "*It is complicated where I live. It is 44 km* [and] *It is tough in winter; it is loads of mud ... If people get sick, they have to be brought in on hammocks ... and it takes a lot of time*" (Rodrigues *et al.* 2021). Importantly, healthcare is not simply a case of opting for either traditional or formal routes. "Care practices conform to a hybrid pattern of health system composition, in which the subsystems are activated in an overlapping, non-exclusive, and interactive way according to individual and community needs, and the insufficiency of the responses by the public health system" (Rodrigues *et al.* 2021). There is a "care mosaic" here.

China

The structure of the healthcare system in China was reformed in 2009 into a three-tier system that distinguishes rural and urban areas. The tiers in the rural system comprise village clinics, township health centres (THCs), and county hospitals, while the urban system comprises community health centres (CHCs), city and district hospitals and regional hospitals. The 2009 reforms also proposed that at least 90 per cent of the population should have healthcare insurance cover. Currently, 95 per cent are covered by one of two publicly funded medical insurance schemes. In urban areas those employed have to be enrolled in the Urban Employee Basic Medical Insurance (UEBMI) while the Urban Resident Basic Medical Insurance (URMS) is for those residents without formal jobs or the unemployed, including children and older people. The New Rural Cooperative Medical Scheme (NCMS) was established in 2003 for the rural population.

Both URMS and NCMS are voluntary schemes, so some payments are still out-of-pocket. Recent evidence suggests that the take-up of these voluntary schemes has been shrinking because of rising costs of premiums:

> Yuan Lixia, a 45-year-old migrant worker in the southern Hunan province, decided this year to withdraw from the main health insurance policy, which covered less than 40 per cent of a Rmb20,000 ($2,800) back surgery he underwent in March. "The insurance hasn't done much to ease my medical burden ... I might as well spend more money on high-quality food to stay healthy".[8]

Yu and colleagues (2021) have examined the distribution of doctors (general physicians) across the Chinese provinces (Figure 5.5). Table 5.2 shows those provinces with the lowest and highest provision of doctors per head of population, but also by area, in 2018. Clearly, there is reasonably equitable provision according to population but large and sparsely populated provinces such as Inner Mongolia have a very low density of coverage. As the authors put it: "China's high-quality medical resources are mainly concentrated in large hospitals of eastern cities" (Yu *et al.* 2021: 6). They propose an expansion of digital healthcare (telemedicine) as a possible solution to access difficulties.

8. www.ft.com/content/0ef68e30-bbe7-4b6e-8d17-479a552be994

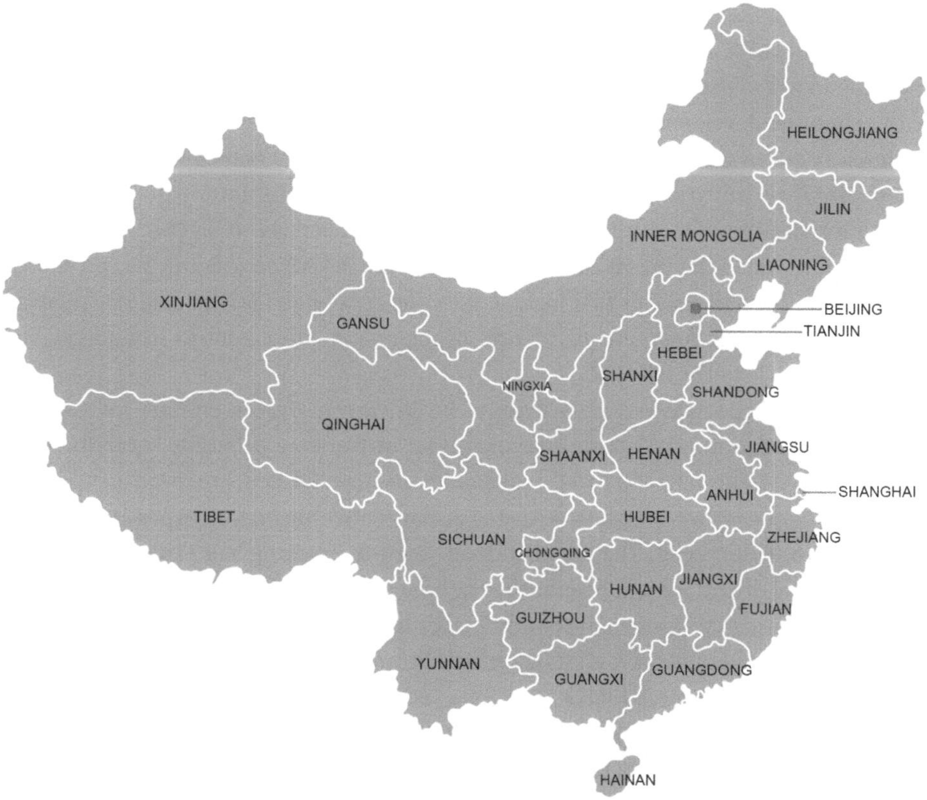

Figure 5.5 Chinese provinces
Source: Gatrell (2023: 35).

Table 5.2 Provinces in China with the lowest and highest ratio of doctors per 1,000 population

Province	*Doctors per 1,000 population*	*Doctors per 1,000 per km²*
Jiangxi	1.88	0.52
Anhui	2.01	0.91
Yunnan	2.06	0.25
Guangxi	2.15	0.45
Gansu	2.26	0.13
Beijing	4.63	5.94
Zhejiang	3.33	1.87
Shanghai	2.95	11.29
Inner Mongolia	2.90	0.06
Jiangsu	2.90	2.27
China average	2.62	1.33

Source: Yu *et al.* (2021).

Qin *et al.* (2024) examine the geographical distribution of medical resources (the number of doctors and hospital/clinic beds, per million population) across 290 cities, using data for the first two decades of the twenty-first century. These data are correlated with economic development statistics (including GDP). The variation across all cities declined between 2010 and 2020, suggesting an increasingly equitable distribution of resources. In a positive conclusion they "are confident that in the future, the unequal distribution of healthcare resources in China will gradually decrease" (Qin *et al.* 2024: 17). As evidence, they note that the Healthy China Action (2019–30) programme has promoted economic and health policies that include the construction of national regional medical centres; 125 projects for the construction of regional medical centres in underserved provinces were listed in July 2023.

Song *et al.* (2024) base their analysis of healthcare resources on data for Chinese counties and examine the within-province level of resource provision; over the time period 2002–11 the overall spatial inequalities of hospital bed provision in counties improved significantly. Nevertheless, spatial disparities within provinces persisted. While six provinces (Chongqing, Tianjin, Shandong, Jiangsu, Zhejiang and Hainan) showed a relatively equal distribution of hospital beds, three others (Xinjiang, Inner Mongolia and Qinghai Province; see Figure 5.5) showed higher levels of inequalities.

In an ambitious study Jia *et al.* (2022) describe and analyse spatial accessibility to all primary healthcare centres (PHCs) in China, assembling data both for PHC locations and community populations on a 100 m × 100 m grid. Over 55 per cent of the 4 million communities (representing about 70 per cent of the total population) had at least one PHC within their 6 km catchment areas. Inevitably, the shortest distances were in the main cities and the longest were in western provinces; however, there is considerable within-province variation in distance travelled from communities to PHCs. The authors go on to use the enhanced 2SFCA method (above, pp. 18–19) to calculate the spatial accessibility of each community. Since the main urban areas are more densely populated than western provinces they reveal better accessibility than the latter. However, the authors assume the same service characteristics in every PHC. They acknowledge that "large variation in overall capacity may exist" and that "more local work needs to be done to identify the actual access at the household level [since] non-spatial factors could affect spatial accessibility as well, such as quality of care in PHCs" (Jia *et al.* 2022: 9, 11).

More locally, Wang *et al.* (2018) examined the provision of healthcare in Sichuan province, one of the largest (by population and area; Figure 5.5) but also one of the more heterogeneous, with an urban south-east and a rural, less-developed north-west. As they say, "Sichuan serves as a microcosm of the broader situation in China" (Wang *et al.* 2018: 22). Their work deals only with primary care (provided by CHCs and THCs); given the SE/NW "divide" it is understandable that this is mirrored by unequal access to primary healthcare. In the west near the Hengduan mountains people may live over one hour from their nearest THC, while near Chengdu (the provincial capital) most are within half an hour from the nearest CHC. Further, a large proportion of the population in the north comprise not the country's majority Han ethnic group but minority groups, including Tibetan.

Traditional Chinese Medicine (TCM) embraces a number of practices, including acupuncture, tai chi and herbal medicines, many of which are, of course, widely used outside China. Lu and Zeng (2018) suggest that demand for TCM in China is "immense" and note that the number of those using TCM hospitals increased from 170 million in 2009 to 471 million in 2014. Within China itself there is a variety of complementary and alternative practices, not least those involving ethnic groups in the west and north of the country: Uighurs, Tibetans and Mongolians (Yu & Amri 2016). With this caveat in mind Xu *et al.* (2022) have explored the geography of TCM, noting that a TCM Development Plan (2016–30) has strengthened its importance as part of overall healthcare provision in China. Geographically, Inner Mongolia, Gansu and Beijing (all in the north of the country) had the best provision of TCM centres, bed numbers and staff, per head of population, in 2019.

Increasing life expectancy and previous limits on family size (now all removed) have led to a rapidly ageing population. Currently, about 15 per cent of the population is aged over 65 years and this is projected to rise to 25 per cent by 2035.[9] How does this impact on access to healthcare?

Drawing on data from several waves of a longitudinal survey of adults aged over 65 years Zhang *et al.* (2017) show that while reported access to healthcare was generally high among those surveyed, older adults living in rural areas were almost twice as likely as those in urban areas to report poor access to healthcare. As they reveal, this has implications for health outcomes. They suggest that older people in rural areas who have traditionally relied on family members for care find that this has lessened as young family members have migrated to urban areas, whether for education or work. Again, there appears to be a clear east–west divide. As Mai *et al.* (2022: 6) put it:

> the advanced and excellent healthcare resources are mainly distributed in the eastern region of China, followed by the central region, while the western region is relatively insufficient. The unbalanced healthcare resources distribution hinders older adults who are living in remote areas from getting immediate or enough healthcare services.

Lin *et al.* (2023) note a reluctance among older people to access healthcare. Most rural Chinese adults managed their illnesses themselves, and results from their study (interviewing 108 older adults from 12 villages close to a city in southern China) found people using herbal medicines or food to cope with illnesses. While they had sufficient

9. www.eiu.com/n/

time to use available healthcare resources, their attitudes towards seeking medical care were negative. "Influenced by the traditional culture and closed social environment, rural older people gave little weight [to] doctors' advice, and adopted a variety of informal self-treating" (Lin *et al.* 2023: 7). As one interviewee put it: "*I am too old, so I don't want to go to the hospital. It is very troublesome and time-consuming there, and the queues are very long. It might take me a whole day just to get an examination done*".

As noted in an earlier chapter it is important to measure access to primary care in order to assess whether better access puts less pressure on secondary (hospital) services. From a geographical perspective the same applies to *spatial* accessibility. Chen and Pan (2022) have explored this in one city, Chishui (in northern Guizhou province) using data for 2014–17. They find that spatial accessibility to primary care facilities is inversely related to potentially avoidable hospitalization, suggesting that improving the former would reduce the latter. In addition, they note that once spatial accessibility is controlled for, those in poorer households or living in less affluent areas were more likely to be hospitalized; they suggest that this might be explained by lower levels of health literacy, or poorer self-management of health issues.

In a short section on health inequalities in China (Gatrell 2023: 35–7) I drew attention to the very poor health of the minority Uighur (Uyghur) population in the west. Unequal access to healthcare, and severe maltreatment of that population is no different (Box 5.4).

BOX 5.4 THE NON-HEALTHCARE OF THE UIGHUR POPULATION IN CHINA

While much of this section on China has considered unequal access to primary and secondary healthcare, with a specific focus on spatial accessibility, there is little "care" offered to the Uighur population (living mainly in Xinjiang province); indeed, the very opposite is the case. The United Nations has reports of organ harvesting from Uigurs and others detained in camps. "The most common organs removed from the prisoners are reportedly hearts, kidneys, livers, corneas and, less commonly, parts of livers. This form of trafficking with a medical nature allegedly involves health sector professionals, including surgeons, anaesthetists and other medical specialists".[10] In a *Lancet* editorial Richard Horton refers to evidence of "forced sterilisations, forced placement of intrauterine devices, and forced abortions [which] may have contributed to a rapid fall in the birth rate in Xinjiang" (Horton 2022: 798). Horton criticizes the Director-General of the WHO, Tedros Adhanom Ghebreyesus, for speaking about human rights violations elsewhere but failing to acknowledge the evidence, provided by the United Nations, concerning the Uighur population.

10. United Nations press release, 14 June 2021: www.ohchr.org/en/press-releases/2021/06/china-un-human-rights-experts-alarmed-organ-harvesting-allegations?LangID=E&NewsID=27167

India

India is divided into 28 states (Figure 5.6), each of which has considerable autonomy. The population in 2024 was 1.44 billion. In 2012, according to Dubey *et al.* (2023), when the population was 1.3 billion 23 per cent were living below the poverty line; this of course varies by state, with about 5 per cent in Goa and almost 40 per cent in one of the poorest states, Chhattisgarh.

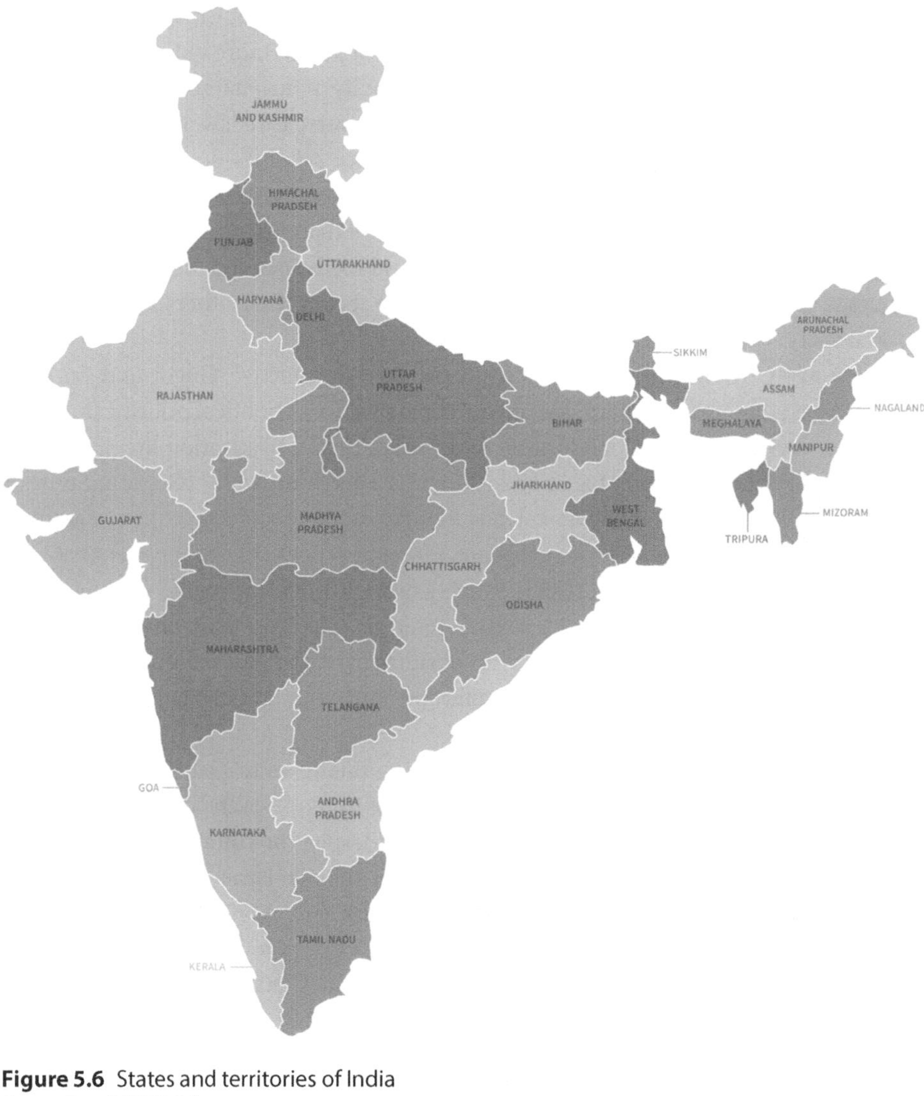

Figure 5.6 States and territories of India
Source: Gatrell (2023: 34).

Healthcare in India is funded by government, private sources and out-of-pocket expenditure and the last of these accounted for about 55 per cent of total health expenditure in 2019, though in 2023 this had reduced to 44 per cent (Dubey *et al.* 2023).

In 2007 India set up the Rashtriya Swasthya Bima Yojana (RSBY), a programme that provides free medical care for poorer people. This was relaunched in 2017 as Ayushman Bharat, with the intention of achieving universal health coverage (UHC); however, states have discretion as to whether they wish to participate in the scheme. Dubey *et al.* (2023) have an excellent overview of these schemes. Studies of RSBY enrolment have suggested that this is worse in remote rural areas and poorer districts, as well as among Indigenous communities and households with a female head. Detailed work in Chhattisgarh (Nandi *et al.* 2018) found that while insurance coverage was higher in more vulnerable districts (those including "low-caste" populations), the availability of hospital services is inversely proportional to vulnerability: a good example of the inverse care law. Importantly, they conclude that "equitable enrolment in health insurance schemes does not automatically translate into equitable access to healthcare" (Nandi *et al.* 2018: 1); that depends on service provision. Moreover, "availability" means more than just the presence of a hospital. As Patil *et al.* (2023) note, shortages of staff and medicines and diagnostic services encourage some people toward the expensive private sector, while others postpone their hospital visits.

Others agree. Writing from a political economy perspective Gogoi and Sumesh (2022) suggest that "insufficient public investment, absence of political prioritization and leadership, and a push for liberalization and unregulated privatization are significant constraints to the realization of accessible and affordable healthcare" (Gogoi & Sumesh 2022: 225). Private sector involvement has increased, and according to these authors accounts for about 80 per cent of outpatient care and 60 per cent of inpatient care. In an excoriating account they assert that "some private hospitals promote various forms of malpractises [*sic*], including unnecessary referrals, needless diagnostic tests, drug prescriptions for paybacks, gifts and travel subsidies from the pharmaceutical industry, unnecessary surgeries and procedures, collusion with organ transplant rackets, and insurance fraud" (229).

There is a shortage of health professionals in the public sector, particularly in rural areas. As a result, marginalized populations lack access to good healthcare and the authors suggest that this has its roots in India's colonial past, despite the country achieving independence more than 75 years ago: "India inherited a colonial legacy and remains elitist and urban-centric in its implementation of public health care policies" (Gogoi & Sumesh 2022: 230).

Turning to geographical constraints, Patil and colleagues (2023) examine how transport difficulties constrain access to healthcare for older adults in the city of Bengaluru (formerly Bangalore), Karnataka state. They interviewed 60 people aged over 50 years and their data provide a rich picture of the realities of getting to healthcare facilities.

Transport was often unreliable, journeys lengthy, and other people often proved unhelpful during the journey, while the Covid-19 pandemic brought additional problems. The cost of transport is a problem for some. Ratna (66 years old) said: "*Not prefer to walk. I have to walk. For every little thing I can't, my medical expense is more ... So, I have to think, whether to spend on auto for little distance or let me walk slowly*" (in Patil *et al.* 2023: 9). There are differences according to income, with some adults insured and others not, and some able to hire a driver and others needing two or more bus trips to access services. Relative location matters too: those living on the outskirts of the city had more trouble getting to clinics, delaying timely access. As the authors conclude: "Providing equitable access to public transport will help older adults be independent and make use of preventive healthcare services for better health outcomes" (Patil *et al.* 2023: 11).

Thakkar and colleagues (2023) note the improvements in maternal mortality made in India over the past 20 years but also that this is geographically patterned, with poorer states (e.g. Assam and Uttarakhand) accounting for most deaths. They examine the extent to which the country meets WHO recommendations for four antenatal visits during pregnancy. In 2015–16 only just over half of pregnant women made such visits. Using survey data for almost three-quarters of a million pregnant women they examined a range of explanatory variables, including both spatial context (region, place of residence: urban/rural, distance to healthcare facility) and individual determinants, including caste. Women living in north-eastern and central states (Figure 5.6) had worse attendance than those in the south. Similarly, those in Scheduled Castes/Tribes had fewer attendances, as did women who reported that distance from healthcare was a factor. In a similar paper using more recent data (2019–21) Girotra *et al.* (2023) confirm the geographical inequality in antenatal visits (Table 5.3) and their data include not only visits but an assessment of the quality of provision (see Figure 5.7, for example).

Table 5.3 Percentage of women with fewer than four antenatal visits, and poor quality of care: worst and best performing states in India

State	*Poor antenatal care*
Bihar	40.61
Nagaland	32.06
Jharkhand	24.90
Uttarakhand	24.24
Arunachal Pradesh	22.80
Goa	0.17
Kerala	1.78
Tamil Nadu	1.90
Puducherry	1.99
West Bengal	3.63

Source: Girotra *et al.* (2023: 7).

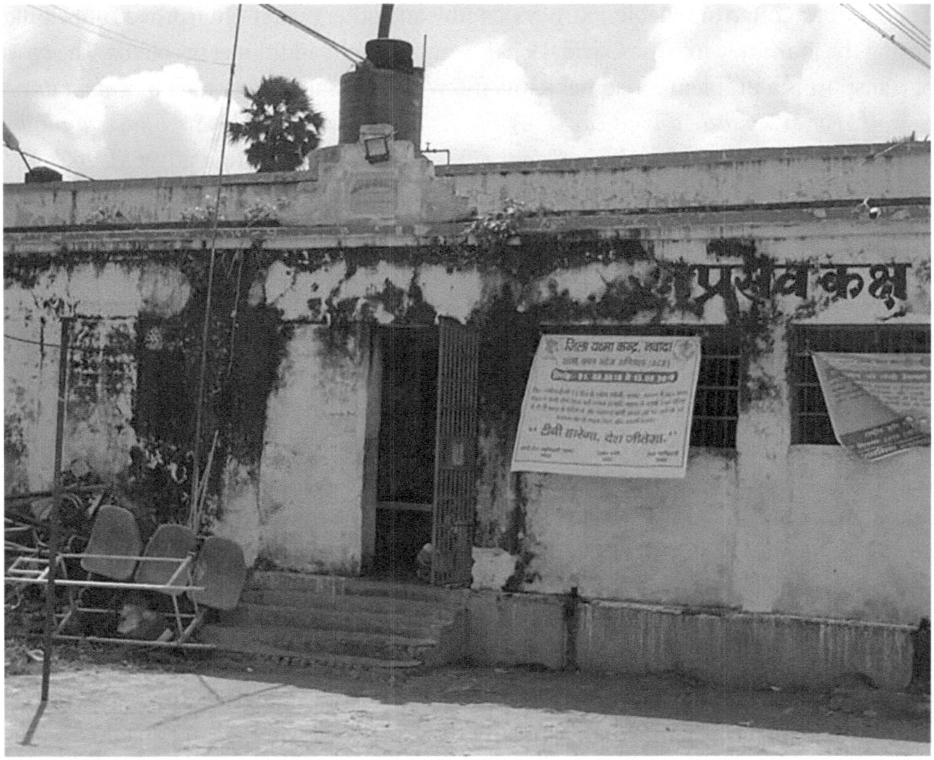

Figure 5.7 A maternity ward in a primary health centre in Bihar (in use until 2019)
Source: www.sylff.org/news_voices/29208/: courtesy of Dr Gautam Anand, University of Oregon.

Given the poor access in some states, instanced in Table 5.3, it is important to delve more deeply into what lies behind this. A key factor is the provision of Accredited Social Health Activists (ASHAs) or female community health workers whose role is to encourage institutional delivery (for which cash incentives are available to expectant mothers). Vellakkal and colleagues (2017) have explored these issues in three states (Jharkhand, Madhya Pradesh and Uttar Pradesh) where antenatal care utilization is low. One factor is the belief that a clinic or hospital delivery is only needed where complications are likely, this leading to delays when such care proved necessary, in which case transport was not always available and women were unable to get to the delivery facility in time. The quality of such facilities is an impeding factor; as one woman put it: "*In hospitals, good doctors are not there. Electricity and water is not always available*".

Others preferred to rely on traditional birth attendants (*dais*). "*The dai has several years of experience. She is taking care of all the delivery in our village. She knows everything. She helps in delivery without much pain by putting oil*". Some ASHAs are critical of hospital facilities:

> *Not many facilities are often available in government hospitals ...* [women] *raise lots of concerns of the quality and often tell us that nurses and doctors will demand money in government hospital ... sometime staff won't be there on holidays and weekends, and night ... for caesarian* [*sic*] *they refer to private hospitals ... and sometime it is difficult to get the ambulance, particularly in the night.*
>
> (all quotes from Vellakkal *et al.* 2017)

Clearly, "access" is a multidimensional issue.

Mozambique

Mozambique gained independence from Portugal in 1975, after almost 500 years as a colony, but this was followed by civil war between competing factions (FRELIMO and RENAMO), and the northern part of the country (Figure 5.8) has suffered for several years from hostile incursions from radical Islamist groups. Healthcare before independence favoured the white population in the cities and sought to protect Portuguese settlers from infectious disease. A third of the healthcare budget in the early 1970s was dedicated to the main hospital in the capital, Maputo, and more than two-thirds of the country's doctors worked in Maputo, mostly in private practice.

Turshen (1999) gives an excellent account of the early post-independence history of healthcare in Mozambique, noting FRELIMO's setting up of broad-based primary care systems. "What is remarkable in the Mozambican story ... is that even in the face of extreme poverty and under the pressure of a destructive guerrilla war, primary health care worked as a strategy to extend health care to formerly underserved populations" (Turshen 1999: 30). However, recent evidence suggests that FRELIMO is losing support, especially among young people. As one commentator observed in early 2025:

> once in power, the liberators forgot where they had come from. The party that promised every citizen a brighter future has now presided for half a century over one of the world's poorest nations. More than half the population, almost 19 million people, live below the poverty line.[11]

The most recent government Strategic Plan ("PESS") for health services refers to having a decentralized system, one that "favours partnerships to maximize the health and well-being of all Mozambicans". Part-funded and supported by USAID and consultants Deloitte, the Plan is very much an aspirational one.

11. www.theguardian.com/commentisfree/2025/feb/06/mozambique-africa-protests-violence-young-voters

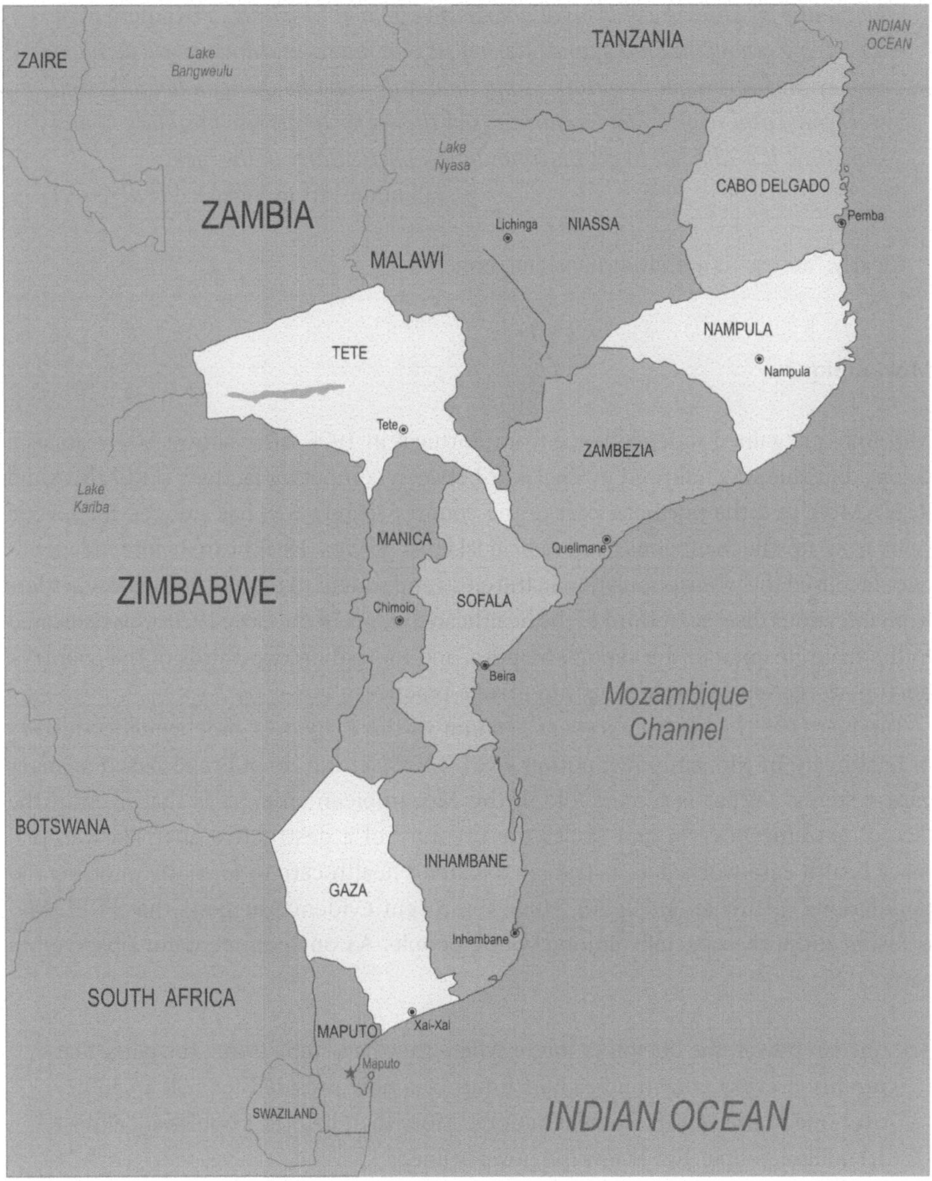

Figure 5.8 Mozambique provinces
Source: Gatrell (2023: 38).

It confirms that the provision involves four types of service provider, as follows:

> The public sector (through the country's National Health System), which has the *widest geographic and technical coverage*. The private sector, which includes for-profit (present mostly in urban areas) and non-profits, represented by national and international NGOs with strong linkages with the public sector. Community level service providers, who partially meet basic needs in areas not reached by the NHS. And lastly, Traditional Medicine Practitioners (TMPs), whose services are widely accepted by communities, complementary to western medicine. [12] (my italics)

We need to unpack some of this provision.

Llop-Gironés and colleagues (2019) used data from the Mozambique Household Budget Survey (conducted in 2014–15: the most recently available dataset) to explore both access to healthcare and the quality of that provided. The data refer to almost 11,500 households and 58,000 individuals and reveal both social and geographic inequality. Those in the poorest household income quintile were least likely to use healthcare services (which could be a community health worker, hospital or traditional healer), while those living in the rural north were significantly less likely to use services than those in the urban south. Those living in the south were more likely to report dissatisfaction with the quality of care given, in terms of waiting times and access to medicines.

But this refers to all healthcare services. What do we know about access to public sector healthcare and its purported "widest coverage"? The national health service in Mozambique has a four-level structure. Community level centres provide basic medical and nursing care while district hospitals offer basic diagnostic, surgical and obstetric care. Provincial hospitals provide more specialist care and workforce training, while there are four tertiary hospitals in the largest cities: Maputo, Beira, Nampula and Quelimane.

Pfeiffer and Chapman (2019) record that in 2011 almost two-thirds of the population lived more than 45 minutes by foot from the nearest health facility, many of which were lacking basic infrastructure, with over half of these lacking access to electricity and clean water. Daca *et al.* (2020), whose research is on child and maternity services, provide a sober assessment of this provision:

> Mozambique is facing critical challenges because of a high burden of disease, a weak health system, a shortage of human resources, deficient management of medical equipment, lack of laboratory consumables and medicines, as well as wide disparities in health outcomes and access to health care within and

12. https://extranet.who.int/countryplanningcycles/sites/default/files/planning_cycle_repository/mozambique/mozambique_-_health_sector_strategic_plan_-_2014-2019.pdf

> between provinces. ... To be vaccinated in Mozambique, the child's mother has to attend a health centre and since 60% of the population lives more than 8 km away from a health facility, transport issues or work load during the harvesting season may impede health care access. (Daca *et al.* 2020: 2)

Clearly, these challenges constrain very severely access to healthcare.

The WHO reported in 2024 on the status of primary healthcare, noting that "various challenges persist in the implementation of the Community Health Strategy (CHS), stemming from a range of factors, such as extreme weather events, including cyclones, floods and droughts, which lead to the internal displacement of people and the disruption of health services". It is argued, rather obviously, that primary care needs bolstering with extra staff and infrastructure: "strengthening this network would increase equitable coverage and access to essential health programs such as routine immunizations and maternal and childcare".[13] Precisely how the WHO expects the country to afford such "strengthening" is not revealed, although one imagines they see a need for private sector and NGO involvement.

On that issue, Pfeiffer and Chapman (2019) have written a highly critical account, suggesting that Mozambique offers "a case study in how the NGO-driven aid model, promoted in tandem with continued austerity in the public sector, undermines progress toward achieving UHC and the SDG goals" and "By the early 1990s, NGOs had multiplied across post-war Mozambique, as the country's adjustment program constrained both public and foreign aid expenditures on the public health system" (Pfeiffer & Chapman 2019: 2). As a result of the imposed structural adjustment policies the proportion of government expenditure fell from 13 to 9 per cent between 2009 and 2015. They conclude that "the Mozambique experience provides an important red flag alerting us to the dangers of the NGO vertical model promoted in tandem with continued [International Monetary Fund] IMF-imposed austerity on public spending" (Pfeiffer & Chapman 2019: 5). Turshen (1999: 38–9) has a similar analysis of the impact of IMF-imposed cuts in expenditure.

Dos Anjos and Cabral (2016) offer a detailed assessment of spatial accessibility, in terms of both walking and driving time, to a large set (over 1,000) of healthcare facilities. Using gridded population data, road network data and elevation they compute both driving and walking distances to such facilities and using a maximum distance of 60 minutes they map those areas that may be classified as underserved (Figure 5.9).

It would seem most useful to consider the walking scenario since few will have access to motorized vehicles, especially in rural areas. Analysis suggests that two-thirds of the

13. https://www.who.int/news-room/feature-stories/detail/strengthening-primary-health-care-with-a-community-health-strategy-in-mozambique

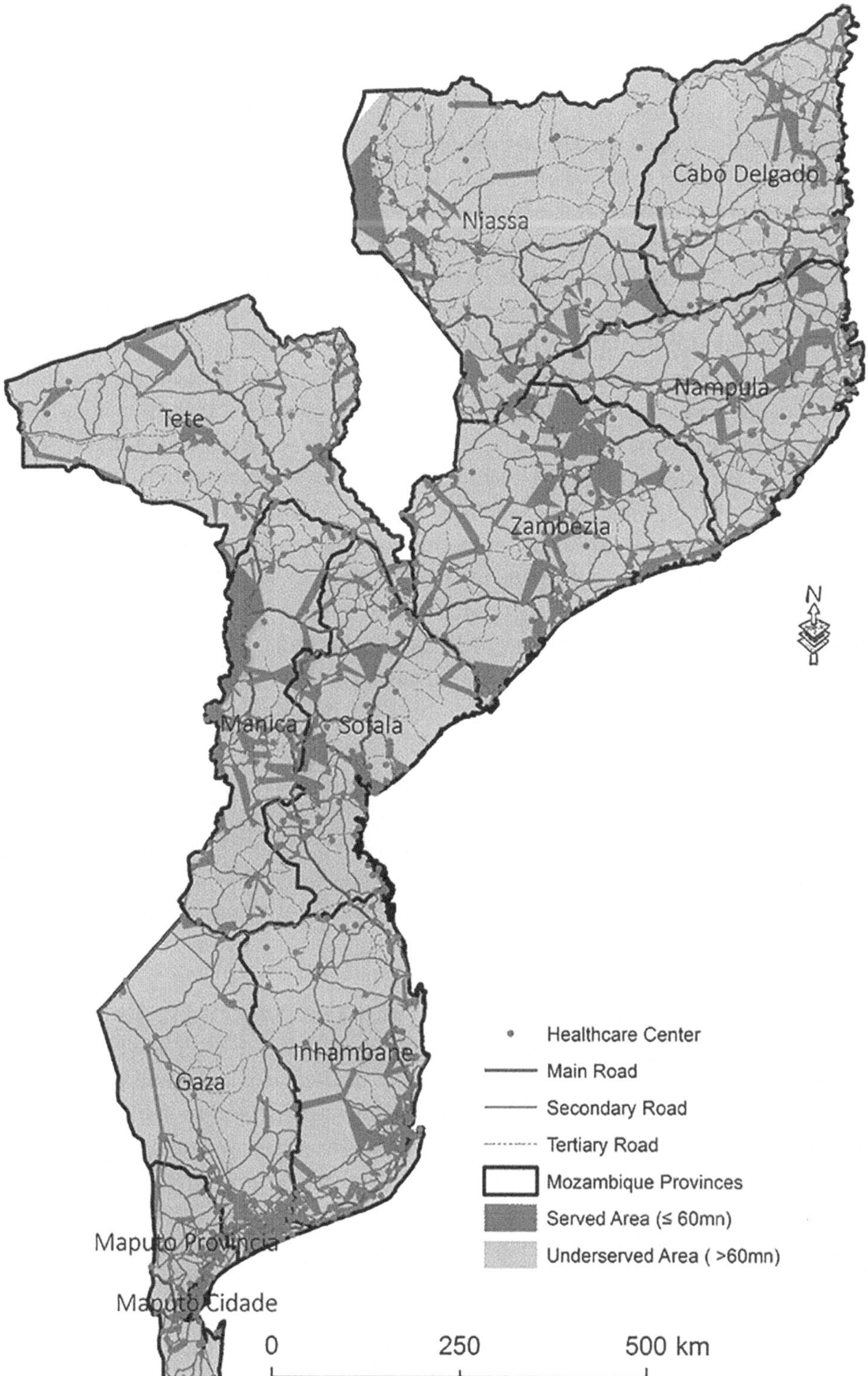

Figure 5.9 Served and underserved areas in Mozambique, by walking time (60 minute threshold)
Source: dos Anjos and Cabral (2016).

population are therefore "underserved", notably in the provinces of Nampula, Zambezia and Tete. As the authors note, there is an assumption in this work that patients travel to the nearest healthcare facility, while some will choose (or have the means) to bypass that and use facilities that may provide better quality services. Further, environmental conditions may constrain travel, certainly by road.

Such environmental determinants have been explored by Petricola *et al.* (2022) and Stone *et al.* (2020). The former considers the impact of flooding caused by Cyclone Idai in 2019 which destroyed or damaged at least 45 health centres; the hardest hit regions were in central Mozambique. Where services are inaccessible there will of course be knock-on effects on disease incidence. By focusing on potential weak points in the road network (those most affected by the flooding) they suggest that up to 10 million people probably experienced worse access to healthcare services. Aside from extreme events such as cyclones there are seasonal impacts on spatial accessibility. Stone *et al.* (2020) found that, between 2012 and 2019, the rainy season has a negative impact on visits for antenatal care, especially for institutional deliveries, and in most provinces. The significant reduction in hospital births is due less to women's choices and more to their not being able to reach the health facility in time. They forecast that in 2021 over 26,000 women who might have delivered in a hospital would not do so during the rainy season. They suggest that for antenatal care there could be better provision of mobile clinics (see later, pp. 150–3) but these will not solve the issue of poor access to institutional facilities for supervised births. As one woman in Zambezia province put it:

> *Access to health care is a big problem. I left my home this morning to reach here. We have a small clinic, but they don't do blood tests. Sometimes we have transport, but today because of the rain it was difficult. It takes about 3 hours to walk, more if you are sick.* (Stone *et al.* 2020: 7)

Where geographical accessibility is limited, traditional healers may be the only form of healthcare for many, particularly those living in rural areas. Takeyama *et al.* (2022) suggest that concerns about the effectiveness of medical treatment and poor spatial accessibility contribute to seeking out traditional medicine. Their in-depth interviews in Pemba city, in Cabo Delgado province, provide an interesting perspective on the latter, known as *curandeirismo* and whose healers (*curandeiros*) draw on medicinal herbs, "divination and magic". Such traditional medicine is respected and trusted by people, regardless of their educational level or social status. One interviewee said: "*I lost confidence in the hospital. I don't think coming back to the hospital anymore. I select an alternative as a curandeirismo*" (Takeyama *et al.*, 2022: 9). As the authors suggest, "people chose treatment from faraway traditional healers rather than nearby medical facilities".

Democratic Republic of the Congo

The Democratic Republic of the Congo (DRC) has a troubled history and a troubled present. Treated in the late nineteenth century as the personal property of King Leopold of Belgium the country achieved independence from Belgium in 1960, suffering both under the dictator Mobutu until 1997 and subsequently because of war and civil conflict in the 1990s, involving neighbouring Rwanda. Mineral resources (including cobalt, diamonds and gold) have long been a factor in these conflicts, with different armed groups seeking control of the mines – many of which are now owned by China.

More recently, during 2023–24, conflict in the north and east (North and South Kivu provinces; Figure 5.10) has led to huge population displacement in the east: up to 7 million people have been displaced since 1996 and as many killed during the same period.[14] The consequences of this for healthcare are discussed more fully in Chapter 6.

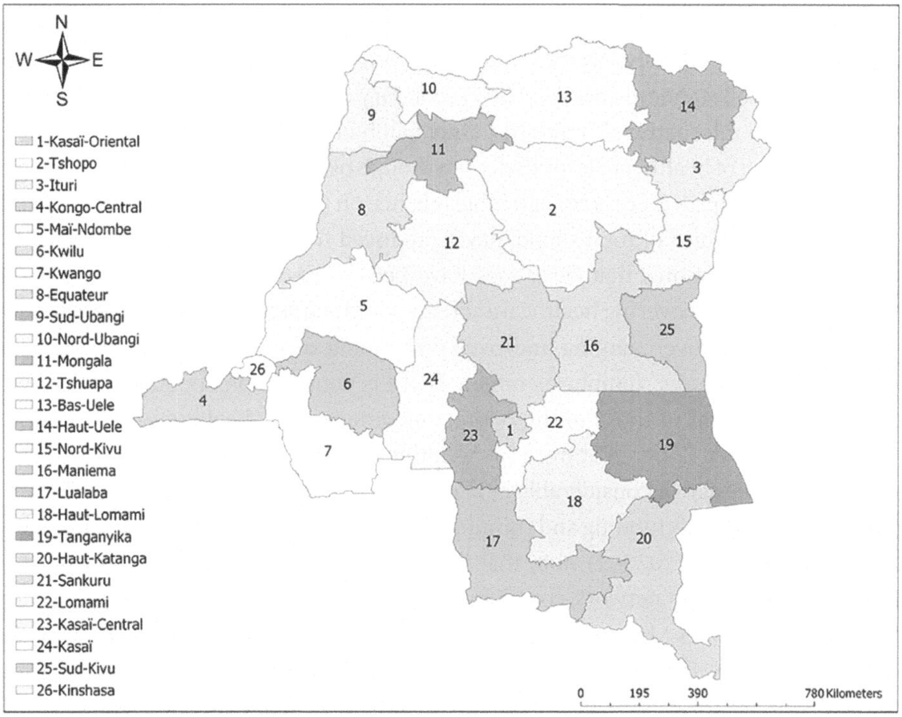

Figure 5.10 Provinces in the Democratic Republic of the Congo
Source: Gatrell (2023: 41).

14. www.cfr.org/global-conflict-tracker/conflict/violence-democratic-republic-congo, dated 21 February 2014.

The country is divided politically into 26 provinces and, further, 516 "health zones" (responsible operationally for primary care). These are further subdivided into "health areas", each of which contains at least one health centre. At the community level are community health workers ("RECOs"), largely peripatetic volunteers who provide reproductive, maternal and child health (RMCH) care, referring upwards to health centres as required.

The organization "Exemplars in Global Health", part-funded by the Gates Foundation, provides some recent pre- and post-pandemic data on healthcare provision. It records that the DRC has 1.2 health workers per 1,000 population, well below the WHO recommendation of 4.45. Data on the distribution of physicians and hospital beds confirm an unequal geographic distribution. In 2006 there were eight hospital beds for every 10,000 people, and much of this provision was centralized in the capital Kinshasa, where 20 per cent of the population lives.

The DRC ranks 167 out of 204 countries in terms of the measure of universal health care coverage. Total health expenditure is under 5 per cent of GDP, at US$23 per capita, well below the suggested targets of 15 per cent and $86 respectively set in the Abuja Declaration in 2001 and reconfirmed in 2023 (Nyamugira *et al.* 2022 suggest that the figures for DRC are actually lower). Out of 8,300 primary healthcare centres, only 1,000 meet international standards, while of 393 secondary centres only just over 200 are built and equipped to international standards. Only half had adequate water supplies.[15]

Public funding of healthcare is limited, even though ostensibly the country is seeking to improve UHC. Instead, there is considerable reliance on user fees; out-of-pocket expenditure is about one-third of total spend, having reduced from about 90 per cent 25 years ago. Criel (2020: 2) notes that "user fees have become *the main source of income for healthcare providers*, covering healthcare activities and staff remuneration. This situation induced substantial overcharging and over-prescribing of medicines, diagnostic tests, and medical procedures" (emphasis mine). There is considerable inequality here, with fewer than 1 per cent of those in the poorest income quintile having health insurance, compared with over 12 per cent from the wealthiest quintile (Nyamugira *et al.* 2022).

Clearly, user fees are a considerable barrier to healthcare utilization. But the Catholic Church also plays a role, funding and running a large number of health facilities, including hospitals. Criel *et al.* (2020: 2) note that "private faith-based healthcare providers, of which the largest is the network coordinated by the Catholic Church (BDOM: Bureau Diocésain des Oeuvres Médicales), play an important role in healthcare delivery and are in most instances well integrated into the public health system".

In addition to these providers mention should also be made of Mutual Health Organizations (MHOs), a form of social protection; these provide health insurance to those who enrol in it, thereby reducing out-of-pocket contributions and, in principle, improving access to healthcare. However, Criel (2020: 2) asserts that the ability of these to improve

15. https://www.exemplars.health/

the quality and affordability of healthcare remains weak. In terms of external aid Criel (2020: 2) further notes that this "is largely assigned to disease-specific programmes such as the Global Fund to Fight AIDS, Tuberculosis and Malaria, or to a diversity of local projects directly funded by multiple external agencies". In other words, such aid is for "vertical" rather than the "horizontal" support for wider primary care that would pay more dividends.

Maini *et al.* (2014) noted that user fees were, in DRC and other African countries, a response to worsening primary healthcare provision, as countries sought to adapt to constraints on government healthcare budgets. In their words, such fees "sought to improve accountability between providers and communities, as well as provide a sustainable way of improving access to health facilities, health-care utilization and quality of care, while lowering frivolous use of health services" (Maini *et al.* 2014: 2). They explored the subsidizing of such fees by donors (including the UK's Department for International Development) but these failed to have any long-term impacts on service utilization. Turshen (1999: 47–52) documents the failure of user fees in particular African countries to improve access to healthcare.

In North Kivu and South Kivu (Figure 5.10) there is a "two-tier" system of provision, with some health areas benefiting from such subsidies while others do not. As one Medical Officer put it:

> *in the health areas that are supported by a partner, there care is free as the partner pays for incentives, equipment, drugs* [...] *and the community utilizes these facilities. But the centers that are not supported and live on self-funding are almost not utilized* [...] *the population is poor* [...] *people prefer seek for care where facilities are supported.* (Altare *et al.* 2020: 13)

People living in health zones that did not have subsidies travelled (often long distances) to access care – a kind of spillover effect.

Pu and colleagues (2020) have undertaken a spatial accessibility study and also explored a set of possible locations for new healthcare facilities in North Kivu province (see Chapter 2 for a brief summary of the methods). Population data were taken from the WorldPop database, and represented at 100 m grid resolution, while road network, elevation and land cover data were obtained from other sources. The accessibility of each grid square to its nearest hospital was computed according to three transport scenarios: walking, motorcycle and bus. Results suggested that 25, 50 and 44 per cent of the population could reach the nearest hospital within two hours, according to the walking, motorcycle and bus travel scenarios, respectively. Location-allocation analysis further suggested that these percentages would increase by around 10 per cent if a further five hospitals were provided. Needless to say, while this is a valuable technical exercise the prospect of substantial additional provision in a conflict-ravaged region of the country seems very remote.

Other research in DRC has confirmed that spatial accessibility is a significant challenge, because of security concerns, the rainy season, or both. Mukendi *et al.* (2019) have examined the utilization of emergency obstetric care, conducting surveys and interviews in 2014 of health providers working in a sample of over 1,500 health facilities in 11 provinces. Such emergency childbirth care was highly uneven geographically, being more available in the urban areas (such as in Kinshasa province). The monitoring of such facilities is poor, owing to lack of funding and staff who lack motivation (and pay). They write: "The health sector is characterized by public underfunding, the uncontrolled production of doctors and nurses, in association with the under-production of qualified midwives. The health infrastructure is insufficient and outdated, and the functioning of health facilities is essentially ensured by patients' payments" (Mukendi *et al.* 2019: 3). This of course has knock-on effects for maternal mortality.

Concluding remarks

There are several important themes threading through this chapter. The first is to remind ourselves that history – particularly that of colonialism – has shaped healthcare provision and delivery. Colonial powers, whether in parts of Africa, or in India, dictated that investment in infrastructure was spatially concentrated. As Turshen (1999: 56) says, such "uneven development meant that the districts with the poorest people could provide only the poorest services". The legacy of colonialism does, in some cases, continue to shape access to healthcare services.

Second, we have noted the enduring and insidious impact of neoliberal policies, especially the World Bank's structural adjustment programmes, where controls on government spending have worsened access to healthcare. We considered this in detail in the case of Mozambique. Yet it is not only the programmes pursued by international organizations that affect access to healthcare in the Global North. It is clear from President Trump's policy initiatives that US reduction, or discontinuation, of healthcare programmes will have very serious impacts on such access and, consequently, on morbidity and mortality. USAID had a budget of $63 billion in 2023 (about 1 per cent of the federal budget) but the 2026 budget proposes cuts of more than 80 per cent, with the charity Oxfam suggesting that "as many as 95 million people would lose access to basic healthcare, potentially leading to more than 3 million preventable deaths per year".[16]

I have chosen to examine healthcare provision and utilization in some detail in five countries in order to illustrate the geography of access in parts of the Global South. In doing so it became clear that some of the particular *geographical* constraints are not so

16. www.oxfamamerica.org/explore/issues/making-foreign-aid-work/what-do-trumps-proposed-foreign-aid-cuts-mean/

different from those in the Global North. How far people live in relation to healthcare facilities is the same issue, even if these distances are often far greater in many parts of the Global South.

Further reading

There is a wealth of literature relating to accessing healthcare in many countries of the Global South and, inevitably, I have been very selective. If interested in a specific country or region then a search on PubMed is recommended.[17]

The classic geographic treatment of healthcare (and health) in the Global South is Phillips (1990) and while this is inevitably dated it deals with access to and accessibility of primary and secondary care, with attention to both provision and utilization.

On UHC the WHO has useful fact sheets.[18]

Although over 25 years old, Turshen (1999) is essential reading for understanding African health systems and especially the role of privatization. In particular, she has important sections on Mozambique as covered above, but also Zimbabwe, Malawi and Zambia. In Chapter 5 she offers a critical account of the role played by non-governmental health services (NGOs).

17. pubmed.ncbi.nlm.nih.gov/

18. See https://www.who.int/news-room/fact-sheets/detail/universal-health-coverage-(uhc)

6

WHO CARES IN TIMES OF CRISIS?

> Emergencies are moments when the past rams into the future, where the relationality of events are made clear, and research across disciplinary and organisational registers is essential Herrick *et al.* (2022: 10)

We may define a humanitarian crisis as a set, or series, of events that poses a critical threat to the security, safety and health of communities, where that threat potentially covers a wide geographical area. The "events" may be triggered by geological forces, such as earthquakes and tsunamis, or by war and conflict. We may also think of climate change as a humanitarian crisis, although the timescale of this is much longer than more "acute" events. Regardless, all these lead to population displacement, food insecurity and the spread of infectious disease. Consequently, the human impacts will be devastating and will demand healthcare to alleviate human suffering. Who provides such healthcare, and how, is the focus of this chapter.

We first take a critical look at "humanitarianism", before examining the provision and nature of care delivered in zones of conflict, as a result of disasters, and during epidemics and the Covid-19 pandemic.

Humanitarianism and its critics

Who can object to governments, organizations (philanthropic or clinical) and well-meaning individuals providing help – resources, time – as forms of "aid" in times of crisis, whether these crises arise from "natural" disasters (such as earthquakes) or from outbreaks of infectious disease? There is, for many, a moral imperative to relieve the human suffering that results from these acute episodes. But we can, and should, cast a critical eye on such endeavours and ask whether we should attend more to the underlying *causes* of disasters, some of which result from the violence (whether physical or structural; see above p. 25) inflicted on populations. We might separate out from such a critique the disasters that result from the earth's physical forces, although even here we can question the humanitarian impulse that responds to acute episodes (flooding for example) that are probably a result of climate change, where the underlying causes of this are far removed from those incurring its costs.

The independent think-tank Humanitarian Practice Network questions a knee-jerk response to critical incidents:

> Just because humanitarian crises are growing in scale and scope it does not mean that international humanitarian assistance is necessarily the right kind of help needed for affected countries. The traditional model of humanitarian response is large international agencies scaling up the sectoral assistance they provide directly to affected populations; this is increasingly ill-suited to many of today's crises.[1]

Put simply, justice matters as much as compassion, human rights as much as emotional responses. Consequently, while exploring below how care can be given, we need to explore the "upstream" factors (of which poverty and inequality are the main culprits) that shape the crises that result. While disasters of course require immediate intervention there needs to be a longer-term focus on addressing inequality; the temporal scales are wildly different.

In their analysis of Covid-19, to which we return below, Herrick and colleagues (2022) refer to two aspects of humanitarian intervention. One is the "moral imperative to intervene on distant suffering" (855), a focus on immediate needs; the other is the global mobility of aid workers that, in the present context, can deliver healthcare. In terms of the former the authors remind us that the humanitarian "gaze" should give as much attention to the marginalized in the Global North as to those living in war zones or refugee camps. In terms of the second aspect, Covid-19 required healthcare in countries of the Global South to be delivered as much by local workers as by international healthcare workers. Chapter 7 considers the balance between the global mobility of healthcare workers and the care that might be delivered by local actors.

Care during conflict

As well as having drastic effects on the health of both combatants and civilians, armed conflict has a set of indirect effects that include destruction of infrastructure (roads, power and water supplies), population displacement and disruption to food supplies. Here, the emphasis is on the impact on access to (both provision and use) healthcare.

1. https://odihpn.org/publication/humanitarian-action-is-the-answer-to-fewer-and-fewer-of-todays-humanitarian-crises/

Collecting data on armed conflict is notoriously difficult but various organizations have sought to compile quantitative indices of the level of conflict, country-by-country. The political geographer Clionadh Raleigh has devised one such index, under the auspices of the Armed Conflict Location and Event Data Project (ACLED). Published biannually, the index "assesses every country and territory in the world according to four indicators – deadliness, danger to civilians, geographic diffusion, and armed group fragmentation – based on analysis of political violence event data collected for the past year".[2] In January 2024 the following countries registered "extreme levels" of conflict: Myanmar, Syria, Palestine, Mexico, Nigeria, Brazil, Colombia, Haiti, Yemen and Sudan. This set helps in part to motivate the choice of conflict settings below, in which we examine healthcare responses.

As a generalization, in fragile states characterized by armed conflict, "healthcare provision is configured by multiple actors beyond the reach of a state absent, unwilling or unable to provide public services" (Hill *et al.* 2014: 2). Provision is characterized by both non-government and private sector actors (frequently operating in an uncoordinated way), but also agencies operating across borders. On the latter issues of "mobilities" (to which we return in the following chapter) Hill *et al.* (2014: 4–5) assert that "With porous territorial borders, massive movements of people, ideas, goods, fighters, weapons, health workers, aid agencies, resources, medicines and diseases follow". The search for healthcare across borders has been reviewed by Baatz *et al.* (2022: 1) who refer to this as "therapeutic geographies": "the tendency of healthcare to geographically reorganize within and across borders, specifically under conditions of war". (This is not to be confused with the widely used concept of "therapeutic landscapes": above, p. 9).

Haiti provides a distressing example, with much of the capital, Port-au-Prince, controlled by gangs whose violence engenders poor access to healthcare, as well as food shortages. Healthcare workers there face considerable risks. Belt *et al.* (2024) report results from their survey of medical students and health workers in Haiti, suggesting that almost half reported that a colleague had been kidnapped in the previous two years. One 26-year-old doctor says: "*When I am in Port-au-Prince, I do not let people know that I am a medical doctor because they see doctors as people who make a lot of money. Therefore, we are automatically targeted by the kidnappers*" (quoted in Belt *et al.* 2024: 4). As noted in the case of Nurse Sadia Khan in Chapter 1, simply travelling to the hospital or health centre involves serious risks, with healthcare delivery obviously impeded if staff are unavailable. The same issues of mobility apply to those seeking healthcare. For example, women travel from Port-au-Prince to give birth in the relative safety of Cap-Haitien on the northern coast of the country. There, obstetrician Dr Mardoche Clervil said "*we have enough beds and staff ... but quite often the patients just can't reach us, either because of their socio-economic problems or because of the violence*".[3]

2. https://acleddata.com/conflict-index/
3. https://www.bbc.co.uk/news/world-latin-america-68602114

Médecins Sans Frontières (MSF) reports in detail on the attacks perpetrated on its facilities. These have included military attacks in countries such as Afghanistan, Syria, Yemen and the Central African Republic (CAR), but staff have also been caught up in inter-community violence. In CAR *"Armed men have stopped our ambulances in the street, threatened our staff at gunpoint, and pulled out the patient in back of the ambulance and taken them away, denying them medical care"*.[4] The International Red Cross works with the Red Crescent movement in the HealthCare in Danger project, "addressing the issue of violence against patients, health workers, facilities and vehicles, and ensuring safe access to and delivery of health care in armed conflict and other emergencies".[5] The appalling situation in Gaza merits particular attention (Box 6.1).

BOX 6.1 CONFLICT IN GAZA

In an important, although now sadly outdated, piece Smith (2015) speaks of the "siege" of Gaza, which has for years undergone political domination by Israel that has sought to isolate the Palestinian population living in the territory. His interviews, in 2014, led him to "argue that the data collected indicates that siege impinges on effective healthcare provision through two central, intertwined processes: withholding materials and resources and undermining healthcare at a systems level" (Smith 2015: 333). In terms of the former, there is a lack of medicines and spare parts for equipment; as for the latter, he pointed to a lack of coordination and cooperation in healthcare delivery. Of course, what was a system in crisis has been, from 2023 onwards, systematically destroyed, with healthcare workers killed and healthcare facilities bombed. A number of reputable sources provide the evidence, among which I draw on MSF. The organization notes – as did Smith – that the healthcare system in Gaza was in crisis well before Hamas's attack in October 2023, because of the Israeli blockade. They report that, in May 2024, 24 hospitals have ceased to function and almost 500 healthcare workers have been killed.[6] The World Health Organization reported in May 2025 that only 19 of the 36 hospitals in Gaza remained operational.[7] Dr Qandil, an emergency physician at one functioning hospital (Nasser Medical Complex, Khan Younis, southern Gaza) reported as follows:

> What we are seeing as healthcare professionals is indescribable and devastatingly catastrophic. Even at the most basic level we are struggling – some days we are working hungry because we have no access to food. On those days the hospital might be able to spare some vegetables to eat in the evening. Of

4. www.msf.org/attacks-medical-care-depth
5. https://healthcareindanger.org/hcid-project/
6. www.msf.org/strikes-raids-and-incursions-seven-months-relentless-attacks-healthcare-palestine
7. https://www.who.int/news/item/22-05-2025-health-system-at-breaking-point-as-hostilities-further-intensify--who-warns

> course, we must remember that this is the situation inside the hospital, where there remains some access to electricity and fuel. Outside of the hospital, the situation is much worse. (Qandil 2024: 272)

Engebretsen and Baker (2024: 1) refer to "Israel's systematic destruction of healthcare infrastructure". More specifically: "Since 7 October, at least 22 hospitals, 51 primary healthcare centres and 59 ambulances were destroyed, and a staggering 565 medical workers, including 106 doctors, were killed. By 20 December, not a single hospital in Gaza was fully functional" (Engebretsen & Baker 2024: 2). BBC News reported that UN agencies have postponed emergency polio vaccination in northern Gaza because of "intense Israeli bombardments, mass displacement and lack of access".[8]

Volunteer doctors travelling from the UK and working for MAP (Medical Aid for Palestine) report similar distressing stories. One, Dr Ana Jeelani, has contrasted the British government's attitude to Gazan patients with its care for Ukrainian refugees. "*I work in a [hospital] Trust [in Liverpool] that openly accepted Ukrainian refugees and provided them with cancer care, NHS care, and we have been told that we cannot accept patients from Gaza*". Another doctor, a surgeon from London told the reporter that "*there were plenty of patients who died because we didn't have appropriate specialists or medications or equipment*".[9]

In March 2025 the UN Human Rights Commission asserted that the attacks on healthcare in Gaza amounted to genocidal acts.[10]

Access to healthcare in the Democratic Republic of the Congo (DRC) was discussed in Chapter 5 but that rather glossed over the issue of armed conflict. As part of a wider study of inequitable access to primary care in four conflict-affected fragile states (Nigeria, Mali, Cameroon and DRC) Ramadan *et al.* (2021) find that, in DRC, women with no education (or low incomes) who live in neighbourhoods that are close to zones of medium or high levels of conflict reported more barriers to access that were both geographical and financial than did women with secondary or further education (and higher incomes). Living close to organized violence exacerbates both wealth and educational disparities in access to primary care services. But how does this potential access translate into revealed access – healthcare utilization?

Altare *et al.* (2020) suggest that, despite the periodic conflict in North and South Kivu (Figure 5.10) there has continued to be provision of child and maternal

8. https://www.bbc.co.uk/news/articles/c3e8j5lv1ygo
9. https://www.theguardian.com/world/2024/oct/07/postapocalyptic-uk-volunteer-surgeons-reflect-on-time-in-gaza
10. www.ohchr.org/en/press-releases/2025/03/more-human-can-bear-israels-systematic-use-sexual-reproductive-and-otherhttps://www.ohchr.org/en/press-releases/2025/03/more-human-can-bear-israels-systematic-use-sexual-reproductive-and-other

healthcare, certainly in the period they study (2017–18). "The prolonged effort by non-governmental organizations and UN agencies to respond to humanitarian needs was likely key in maintaining intervention coverage despite conflict" (Altare *et al.* 2020: 2). Interestingly, they suggest that some armed groups assist those delivering healthcare, for example by helping with the transport of staff and drugs, although hardly for altruistic reasons as they themselves benefit. As a consequence, "coverage of basic preventive schedulable child and maternal health services tend to be relatively high in North and South Kivu, and appears generally better than in many other non-conflict-affected provinces in DRC" (Altare *et al.* 2020: 14). This study contrasts with more recent reports from Amnesty International that paint a more sobering picture. "Widespread checkpoints manned by armed groups, and other deliberate movement restrictions imposed by both government forces and armed groups in Ituri, Sud-Kivu and Nord-Kivu, prevented communities from accessing vital assistance such as food, water and healthcare".[11]

What happens to healthcare in the aftermath of conflict? Both Iraq and Afghanistan provide compelling examples.

Until about 1980 Iraq's health system was among the best in the Middle East but subsequent conflict, notably the Gulf War in 1991 that followed Saddam Hussein's invasion of Kuwait and the US-led invasion in 2003 to remove him from power, damaged infrastructure and has led to many skilled healthcare workers leaving the country. Estimates suggest that between 2003 and 2007 about 18,000 doctors left the country. Webster (2011: 864) notes that "the US-led occupation of Iraq triggered a wave of violence described by the International Committee of the Red Cross (ICRC) as catastrophic for healthcare in the country; conditions for health workers remain grim throughout southern and central Iraq". For some, it was worse than "grim", with the Iraq Medical Association suggesting that up to 2,000 doctors had been murdered. Such shortages are regionally patterned. For example, MSF describes the situation in Hawijah district of Kirkuk (one of 19 governorates), where doctors have either left the country or moved to safer areas:

> Rural primary health-care centres continue to report shortages of medical personnel, drugs, and services. Basic components of hospital medical care, including infection control and nursing skills, are sorely lacking and still in need of external support. The 116-bed district hospital remains without adequate human resource capacity to sustain the availability of emergency surgical services. (Fernandez & Boulle 2013: 901)

11. www.amnesty.org/en/location/africa/east-africa-the-horn-and-great-lakes/democratic-republic-of-the-congo/report-democratic-republic-of-the-congo/

Taniguchi *et al.* (2021) offer a more up-to-date picture, examining regional variations in the level of out-of-pocket healthcare expenditure that is described as "catastrophic" (which they describe as amounting to more than 10 per cent of household expenditure). Among the governates, the level of such catastrophic health expenditure ranged from about 9 per cent in Baghdad to 21 per cent in Kirkuk and only a little lower in two other northern governates (Duhok and Erbil – like Kirkuk, oil-rich regions). Some years after the conflicts suffered in the country there remain widespread regional inequalities.

One writer refers to "the toxicity of Iraq's post-2003 patchwork public and private healthcare system" that binds together a set of unscrupulous actors (hauliers, doctors, pharmacists, politicians, drug companies) into a network that compromises the health of people seeking medicines:

> The story of moving medicine ... is a supply chain which is central to the conflict and violence within Iraq and has harmed many more of its citizens than the direct violence which often catches the attention of policymakers. For many Iraqis, their country is not "post-conflict", despite being labelled as such.[12]

In Afghanistan the emergence of the Taliban government in 2021 and the withdrawal of international donor support has compromised the healthcare system. The restriction of rights for women and girls by the Taliban is well-known and this has had serious consequences for nursing provision, as these professionals have seen opportunities for education removed and, according to the International Council of Nurses, many have left the country (Tao *et al.* 2023). Restrictions on women's movements (such as the requirement for a male chaperone or "*mahram*" to accompany them to appointments) have affected their access to healthcare. Expectant mother Nasrin was delayed by Taliban checkpoints for several hours on her way to hospital in 2024 because she was unaccompanied by a male relative; as a result, both she and her baby died.[13] If girls are denied a secondary or higher education, and women can only be seen by a woman doctor, there are obvious consequences for the long-term healthcare of women. While some conflict has ended, a "war on women" seems an appropriate description of the current situation under the Taliban.

Care during natural disasters

There are both short-term and longer-term impacts of natural disasters on healthcare systems. Such disasters will destroy healthcare and related infrastructure that may take

12. www.chathamhouse.org/2022/11/moving-medicine-iraq-networks-fuelling-everyday-conflict
13. https://www.theguardian.com/global-development/2025/apr/03/i-begged-them-my-daughter-was-dying-how-taliban-male-escort-rules-are-killing-mothers-and-babies

years to recover and rebuild. I consider briefly here two examples: the Haiti earthquake of 2010 and that in Myanmar, before turning attention to the impact of Hurricane Katrina on New Orleans in 2005.

The Haiti earthquake caused well over 300,000 deaths and an equivalent number of serious injuries, along with displacing 1.3 million people (roughly one-tenth of the population) from their homes (Figure 6.1).

Hirose *et al.* (2022) document some of the impacts of the Haiti earthquake on access to maternal healthcare, including family planning, antenatal care, delivery and vaccinations. They compare outcomes before and after the earthquake as well as the healthcare outcomes for women directly impacted by the earthquake and those not directly impacted. Their statistical analysis suggests that mothers who lived some distance from the most severely impacted areas experienced as much deterioration of healthcare access as those who lived in the earthquake-affected areas. This may reflect long-standing structural issues affecting the country as a whole; infrastructure was inadequate even before the earthquake hit. These findings are echoed by others. Arnaouti and colleagues (2022) note that, before the earthquake struck, almost half the population lacked access to basic medical care, while almost two-thirds of the country's medical facilities were partially or wholly destroyed. Their review highlights the international response, argued to be the largest humanitarian intervention in a single country, that included military

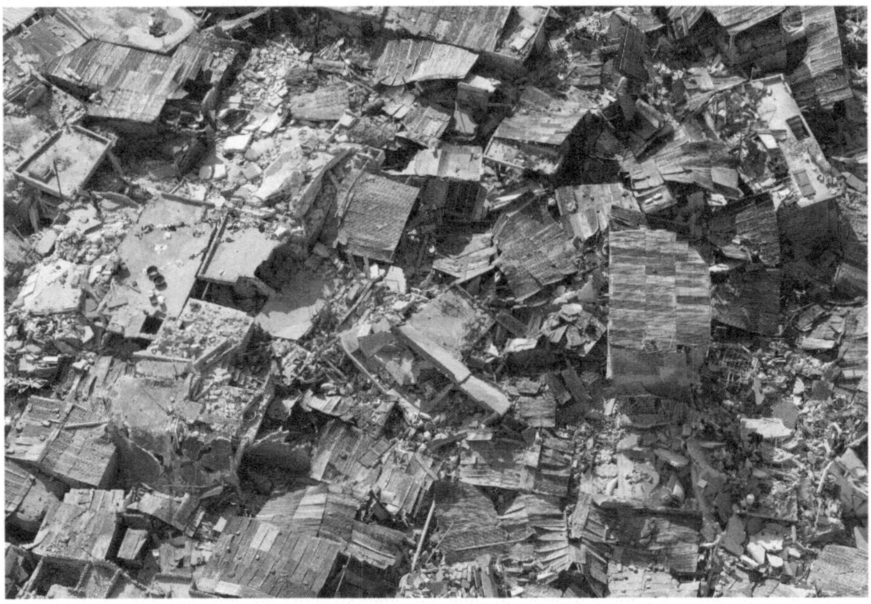

Figure 6.1 Destruction in Haiti as a result of the 2010 earthquake
Source: Wikimedia Commons

help from 26 countries and the involvement of over one thousand NGOs. However, "despite the massive influx of personnel, equipment, supplies, and money, the response was hindered by an inability to manage what resources were available" (Arnaouti *et al.* 2022: 21). Further, there was a lack of engagement with local actors and government and a need to build capacity with them.

Since the devastating 2010 earthquake there have been others in Haiti, albeit with much less loss of life. But outbreaks of infectious disease, notably cholera, have an impact on healthcare. In parts of the capital, Port-au-Prince, armed gangs impede movement, including that of clinical staff, leading to lack of access to healthcare facilities.

The earthquake in March 2025 that devastated parts of Myanmar and killed over 2,700 people has led to accusations that the country's military dictatorship was blocking supplies of emergency healthcare and aid. One Australian doctor, Dr Nang Win, asserted that "aid was confiscated by the military junta", while another doctor, Dr Tun Aung Shwe (and a member of the country's exiled opposition), reported that checkpoints were blocking the flow of medicines to areas that were currently under the control of resistance groups.[14]

In a very different context, hurricanes affecting much wealthier countries can also challenge healthcare delivery. Hurricane Katrina, which caused major flooding in New Orleans in 2005, is a case in point, where almost 1,600 people died and four-fifths of the city was flooded. Iwai *et al.* (2022: e8) assert that "the brunt of Katrina, like COVID-19, was shouldered by Black communities and people of colour who neither received the immediate care nor adequate support in the aftermath". At Memorial Hospital in the city protocols in the event of an emergency were poorly understood, "leading to confusion on which categories of patients should be evacuated first" (e8). Here, as in other cases, there are major ethical issues in determining how to triage people already within healthcare settings such as hospitals.

In terms of longer-term impacts on healthcare, Bell and colleagues (2020) demonstrate that there were significantly fewer primary care physicians in New Orleans five years after the hurricane, although this was not the case for other clinicians. This reflects a wider demographic shift: poorer New Orleans residents remained in the city while those on higher incomes (including higher-earning healthcare providers) left. As the authors note: "Counties affected by Hurricane Katrina already faced socioeconomic disparities; the impact of the storm and its resultant years of recovery undoubtedly exacerbated this" (Bell *et al.* 2020: 8). Sheller (2013: 187) makes a more general point, reminding us that "mobility can be considered a fundamental capability for human thriving, and hence for recovery from disasters". She asserts that "mobility regimes in post-disaster situations bring ... foreign responders and assistance to some of the affected population, while

14. https://www.theguardian.com/world/2025/apr/01/myanmar-earthquake-junta-accused-blocking-aid

holding the 'internally displaced' in place, in an ongoing process of marginalization, serial displacement, and containment – as if they were marooned on an island of misery" (187). Links between mobility and healthcare are considered in Chapter 7.

Care during epidemics: the case of Ebola

Before Covid-19 took all the headlines a different, but also devastating, virus spread across parts of West Africa in 2014–15, in Sierra Leone, Guinea and Liberia in particular. This was Ebola (see Figure 1.2). I have outlined elsewhere the ways in which the disease spread through networks and porous borders (Gatrell 2023: 160–62). Here my concern is less with the epidemiology and more with how care was delivered.

The late Paul Farmer has described this – drawing on his first-hand experience – in a superb book (Farmer 2020) and here I attempt to summarize his basic arguments, the main one being that the (limited) healthcare on offer focused too much on isolating infected patients and preventing further transmission, and less on delivering care to relieve their appalling suffering. In a deeply personal – and angry – account, he records that over one thousand healthcare workers resident in the three countries became infected, and half of them died. This contrasts with Europeans and Americans who became infected, since many were "medevacked out of the clinical desert" (Farmer 2020: xxvi). There was a marked absence of supportive and critical care (intravenous rehydration and possibly blood transfusions), but clinical staff were also understandably wary of themselves being infected. He also suggests that, while primary healthcare needed (and needs) strengthening in West Africa, what was missing was the intensive care facilities that are taken for granted in much of the Global North. Funding to support the creation of these was in scarce supply because of the structural adjustment policies that had been imposed on governments by the World Bank. This meant that these parts of West Africa were both "public health deserts" and "clinical deserts", as Farmer (430) puts it, a feature he attributes to years of colonial rule. Further, earlier armed conflict in both Liberia and Sierra Leone had seriously weakened the healthcare systems such that in one of the latter's districts an abandoned school that had been designated a 108-bed Ebola facility instead "had no walls and seemed more like a bunch of decaying sheds than a permanent structure" (Farmer 2020: 77). A further complicating factor in the provision of healthcare was that people living in these countries were suspicious of the motives and plans put in place by public health officials acting on behalf of governments.

Raven and colleagues (2018) interviewed 25 healthcare workers in four districts within Sierra Leone, some local and others international, documenting their experiences and coping strategies during the outbreak. The key issues that emerged were: the extent to which the health system was prepared to manage the outbreak; its impact on healthcare workers; how they coped; and the various responses to managing the outbreak. On the first of these, one worker drew on a military metaphor: "*You need to have the necessary equipment to fight. What has been the problem is that even when there is this readiness of facing this battle we have not been given the proper equipment to fight*" (in Raven *et al.* 2018: 4). Others were willing to risk their own health and were altruistic: "*We just feel that we are Sierra Leoneans and we should [help], if we do not go into and help our people who will do that?*" (7). This was in the context of almost 400 health workers infected with Ebola in Sierra Leone, of whom 221 died. Since 2016 the number of healthcare providers per head of population has reduced, from 3.4 per 10,000 to 1.4 per 10,000, placing a further burden on the country's healthcare system.

James and colleagues (2020) undertook a similar study, also interviewing healthcare workers in Sierra Leone. The same findings of altruism come out in their study:

> *Well, for me, I took an oath to serve no matter the circumstance, and I cannot see my fellow Sierra Leoneans suffering without doing anything. When I was asked to start screening survivors and provide them with basic care, I started crying because I was afraid. That I will not lie. Nevertheless, I ... started providing care to survivors. I just relied on my basic nursing skills and also my experience in providing care to HIV/AIDS patients.* (quoted in James *et al.* 2020: 1386)

But the quality of care on offer was hampered by a lack of equipment (including personal protective equipment) and medication. Nonetheless, the government sought to provide significant assistance, particularly to Ebola survivors. James *et al.* (2020) draw attention to the Sierra Leone government's Comprehensive Package for Ebola Survivors (CPES) programme, introduced in 2016 (since discontinued) with the aims of ensuring that Ebola survivors were given free access to health and psychosocial care. But those interviewed by James and colleagues suggest that the overall healthcare system needs an overhaul, going well beyond providing care to Ebola survivors.

Kamradt-Scott (2016) has reviewed the role played by the WHO in managing the Ebola epidemic. Noting that the WHO had been widely criticized for its mis-handling of the epidemic he points a stern finger at the national governments that fund it. Farmer himself is critical of the WHO, "weakened over the years by political feuds and funding shortfalls [it] had little operational capacity and was unable to act promptly or effectively" (Farmer 2020: 61).

As we have seen, some research has explored, via interviews, the experiences of healthcare workers who treated Ebola patients. A very personal story of one such worker is given in Box 6.2.

BOX 6.2 AN EBOLA PATIENT'S STORY

Dr Ada Igonoh (now Okoli) was a 28-year-old Nigerian doctor working in a Lagos hospital and found herself looking after a patient who had travelled from Liberia and showed symptoms of Ebola virus that was subsequently diagnosed. He died five days after admission, but in the meantime Dr Igonoh herself developed symptoms and was isolated.

> The first person I met when I got to the isolation ward was a World Health Organization (WHO) doctor, Dr. David Brett-Major. He was the only doctor at the time and he came in to see us at least twice daily, shuttling between the male and female wards. He helped out with cleaning up as well, because the nurses were too scared to enter the ward. I was impressed and touched that he came all the way from Geneva to care for us. Soon after, volunteer doctors started to show up at the ward, running about three shifts daily. Some of the volunteers ran away after a few days. I understand; it could not have been easy staring death in the face.
>
> The only treatments I received were bottles of ORS [oral rehydration salts], paracetamol and vitamin supplements. I drank like my life depended on it. I prayed to God like my life depended on it.
>
> I was discharged 14 days after I was admitted after blood tests for Ebola virus came back negative. That gave other patients hope that they would one day leave the ward too.
>
> I have learned that with the right strategies, tools, and resources, we can stop this epidemic. Containing an outbreak is a collaborative effort. When a case is confirmed, the government must act swiftly to stop the chain of transmission.
>
> (Igonoh 2015: 222)

Stories such as this bring home the personal dimension of healthcare and the key role played by both trained medical staff and volunteers. Interestingly, Dr Igonoh herself acknowledges – as does Paul Farmer – that care is paramount, but while Farmer downplays the need for isolation and containment to prevent the spread of the infection she stresses its importance.

Care during pandemics: the case of Covid-19

We have come across the Covid-19 pandemic in earlier chapters but the focus here is largely on the inequities of access to the vaccines. Access to vaccines "in the community" (for example, their delivery in care homes) is something I discuss in Chapter 8. Elsewhere (Gatrell 2023: 166–72) I have discussed the unequal geographies of Covid, particularly concerning the social geography of the infection.

Privor-Dumm and colleagues (2023: 7) asserted that "engaging countries of all income levels, including both state and non-state actors to co-create a new shared vision of access, equity and justice is an urgent action". COVAX (see Box 6.3) sought to ensure that vaccines were developed speedily and distributed equitably, but the same authors reported that, at the end of 2022, while 69 per cent of people across the world had been given a Covid-19 vaccine that shrank to only 25 per cent in low and middle-income countries.

BOX 6.3 COVAX SCHEME

> Countries themselves have a responsibility for their own health systems, but there is also a role for the global community to facilitate action, particularly where health systems are weak and barriers such as food and housing insecurity, poor air quality, discrimination, lack of jobs and education and persistent healthcare access challenges affect health and willingness to be vaccinated.
>
> (Privor-Dunn *et al.* 2023: 2)

The "global community" did respond with a set of partners to establish the COVAX scheme (COVID-19 Vaccines Global Access). This sought to counter "vaccine nationalism" (the hoarding of vaccines to provide a more-than-sufficient supply to meet a country's own needs) and instead to encourage wealthy countries and vaccine manufacturers to donate vaccines as a means of promoting equity in access. There was an element of self-interest, since the potential loss of imports from the Global South and the risk of new variants of the virus spreading "north" suggested there was an economic case to provide support. Puyvallée and Storeng (2022) make this point strongly, noting also that some countries (such as China) preferred to donate directly to specific countries rather than taking part in COVAX. They suggest that the scheme only delivered half of the two billion vaccines that were promised in 2021, well short of the global overall total of 9.25 billion doses total delivered that year. It seems that vaccine nationalism was still at work. Jesudason (2024: e223) provides a more upbeat and updated account and quotes one of the leading partners in COVAX who asserted that:

> COVAX was the largest and most complex emergency response in the history of global health. It delivered 2 billion vaccine doses to 146 countries, averted the deaths of 2.7 million people in lower-income countries, and for many people around the world, was literally the only dependable source of vaccine supply.

The COVAX scheme closed in December 2023 but the emergence of new variants means that booster vaccinations will continue to be required.

Unsurprisingly, a systematic review of vaccine inequality suggested that "in countries/areas where there are adequate health facilities and infrastructure for the production and distribution of COVID-19 vaccine, access to COVID-19 vaccine is higher" (Bayati *et al.* 2022: 7). Kunyenje and colleagues (2023) have examined such inequality across low-income countries in Africa. Some data from 2022 is presented in Table 6.1. Not shown in the table is Rwanda, which was an outlier in the continent, with more than 70 per cent of its population vaccinated. This reflected considerable pre-planning before vaccines (from Pfizer) arrived. Such planning included the purchase of refrigerators and vehicles to transport the vaccine to health centres, as well as open communication about the vaccine and a clear priority list for those most at risk. It is too simplistic to paint the entire African continent as "vaccine-deprived". Senegal too acted promptly to distribute vaccine, leading Büyüm *et al.* (2020: 2) to lament that "international coverage of the continent ... focused on the assumed inevitable failure of African nations to effectively respond to the pandemic, failures which are often caused by limited resources resulting from colonialism and modern-day imperialism".

There were within-country differences. For example, in Malawi the distribution was concentrated in the towns and cities, despite four-fifths of the population living in rural areas. In part, these variations within low-income countries represented the relative lack of manufacturing capacity and appropriate laboratory storage facilities, but variations in the geographic accessibility of vaccination facilities and political instability were contributing factors while in some rural areas vaccine "hesitancy" played a part, as it did in parts of the Global North.

The political dimension of Covid vaccination comes across very clearly in the case of Palestinians living in occupied territories of Israel. As I noted in Gatrell (2023: 172), by February 2021 30 per cent of Israel's population had received two doses of vaccine, compared with 1 per cent in Palestine. MSF claimed that "you are over 60 times more likely to have a vaccination in Israel than in Palestine". By August 2022 the figures had

Table 6.1 Percentage of the population fully vaccinated against Covid-19, December 2022

Country	*Percentage vaccinated*
Mozambique	56.0
Sierra Leone	40.0
Somalia	35.9
Central African Republic	34.7
Afghanistan	26.1
Niger	20.3
Malawi	18.1
Democratic Republic of the Congo	6.9
Madagascar	6.8
Burundi	<1.0

Source: Kunyenje *et al.* (2023).

changed: 68 per cent of Israeli citizens had received two doses, compared with 35 per cent in the occupied Palestinian territories (OPT). Howard and Schneider (2022) have examined this inequity further. Writing before Hamas's violent incursion into Israel they argue that "despite Israeli officials' claims of inclusivity and their dedication to public health, Israel's vaccination campaign, and its corollary refusal to vaccinate Palestinians in the OPT, reflects a form of maiming that advances Israel's settler-colonial aims" (Howard & Schneider 2022: 266). More recently, the Palestinian scholar Nadia Naser-Najjab (2024; see the summary in Adjerid 2024) has explored in detail the experience of Covid-19 in Palestine. Noting, as others have done, that Israel promoted itself as a world leader in vaccination she argues that the pandemic helped to further exercise control and surveillance of Palestinians. Set against the background of conflict she notes that Israel "actively hampered pandemic measures for Palestinians, through blocking or delaying the supply of vaccines, closing virus testing centres, not providing Arabic language health guidelines, and inadvertently discouraging people from testing" (Adjerid 2024: 462). Given ongoing violence in the OPT one can only wonder how vaccination would be disseminated equitably if/when another pandemic appears.

In the US, Yee and colleagues (2024) used GIS to assess geographic accessibility to almost 132,000 Covid vaccination centres. Three-quarters of the population was within 30 minutes walking time to a site offering the vaccine, and 96 per cent within 30 minutes driving time. Of course, this varies from state to state. Almost all the populations of New Jersey, District of Columbia and Massachusetts were within 30 minutes driving time, while this was about 93 per cent in Wyoming.

In terms of other dimensions of access, the Centers for Disease Control (CDC) continues to provide data on vaccination rates among socio-demographic groups (Table 6.2).

Table 6.2 Covid-19 vaccination coverage, US: percentages receiving at least one dose (by 2024)

Indicator	*Percentage uptake*
Poverty status	
Income > US$75k	85.1
Income < US$75k	79.5
Below poverty level	75.5
Ethnicity	
Hispanic	84.6
White	79.4
Black	82.0
Location	
Urban	83.7
Suburban	81.7
Rural	69.7

Source: www.cdc.gov/COVIDvaxview/interactive/adults.html?CDC_AAref_Val=https://www.cdc.gov/vaccines/imz-managers/coverage/COVIDvaxview/interactive/adults.html

Clearly, there is an association with poverty but it is the urban–rural divide that is particularly striking. In part this mirrors spatial accessibility.

Santangelo and colleagues (2024) draw attention to efforts made in Detroit, where 75 per cent of the population is Black and where vaccination rates in early 2021 were substantially lower than in Michigan as a whole. Private companies were engaged to offer free transport to vaccination clinics, the number of which was expanded to meet demand. Interviews of healthcare stakeholders during the pandemic in 2021 suggested that farming communities were disproportionately affected by the limited vaccination sites in rural settings and that while vaccination rates were in part due to poor access to transport, they were also influenced by "politically motivated scepticism" (Kuehn *et al.* 2022). Stakeholders suggested that mobile clinics were an obvious way of improving vaccination rates among vulnerable rural communities (see Chapter 7).

In England Dolby *et al.* (2022) describe variation in the uptake of vaccination from the date it was first rolled out (December 2020) until August 2021. A large study, based on 35 million adults, revealed clear inequalities in vaccination uptake rates according to sex, ethnic group, socio-economic status, education and area deprivation. Specifically, rates of vaccination were low for older Black Africans and all adult Black Caribbeans, as well as those of Muslim religion. People living in more deprived areas, or in rented accommodation, or with fewer educational qualifications or in a lower socio-economic group all had lower rates of vaccination. This work has been updated to March 2023 (and therefore using data on fourth vaccinations) by the Office for National Statistics (ONS) (Table 6.3).

The findings are much the same as Dolby and colleagues reported. Note in particular the clear gradient by area deprivation. But, as the authors acknowledge, describing these inequalities demands explanation. One possibility is vaccine "hesitancy" (or one might say "refusal") – individual concerns, indecision, uncertainty and doubt; this puts the "blame" on individuals or social groups. Another plausible explanation is a lack of trust in what the government proposed regarding vaccinations and/or what health service officials recommend, if prior experiences of such services have been negative. Both are behavioural explanations but one derives from attitudes and another from prior experience.

In a specific geographic context – rural and coastal eastern England – Nanyonjo and colleagues (2023) interviewed 21 health professionals and lay people about their experiences of Covid vaccination. Exploring the lived experience of the actors involved sheds more light on the barriers to, and enablers of, such vaccination. The particular setting was Lincolnshire, a county with areas of deprivation on the coast and some groups without English language, notably from eastern Europe. Some of the latter who were employed in agriculture "questioned why they needed to put things in their bodies if they had 'never had to take a paracetamol in their lives'" (Nanyonjo *et al.* 2023: 4). But the specific geographic context was an important determinant of whether the vaccine

Table 6.3 Ethnicity, deprivation, occupation and vaccination status in England, 2020–23

	Vaccination status [1]
Ethnicity	
White British	78.1
Indian	59.5
Black Caribbean	52.3
Black African	41.8
Bangladeshi	36.3
Pakistani	34.8
Area deprivation	
Q5 Least deprived	81.5
Q4	78.5
Q3	65.4
Q2	69.9
Q1 Most deprived	63.8
Occupational classification	
Higher managerial, administrative and professional occupations	80.7
Routine occupations	71.4

Note: 1 Age-standardized proportions of people aged over 18 years who continued to four vaccinations, December 2020–March 2023.
Source: www.ons.gov.uk/peoplepopulationandcommunity/healthandsocialcare/healthinequalities/bulletins/coronavirusandvaccinationratesinadultsbysociodemographiccharacteristicandoccupationengland/latest

was adopted or not, as were employment constraints. "There were financial challenges associated with travelling long distances to access routine vaccination centres. The organization of services was such that vaccination clinic hours were not convenient for manual job workers" (Nanyonjo *et al.* 2023: 6). Mobile and pop-up vaccination centres helped overcome some of these difficulties.

There are other dimensions to unequal access during the Covid pandemic, notably the impact that it had on disruption to healthcare. Clearly, with government restrictions in place, and people's worries about contracting Covid, there were likely to be impacts on access to healthcare services. Maddock *et al.* (2022), drawing on a variety of longitudinal studies undertaken between April 2020 and January 2021, explored whether such impacts fell unequally on particular groups in the UK. There was a range of disruptions, including to appointments, prescriptions and surgery. Such disruptions were more likely among older adults, among women and among non-white ethnic groups (particularly Black people). In addition, people working in manual or routine occupations were more likely to experience disruption than those in professional and managerial occupations. The reasons are not entirely clear but could include worries about attending healthcare settings and potential exposure to the virus, and caring responsibilities that inhibited attendance. Inevitably, these disruptions to healthcare will have consequences for subsequent health.

These findings are mirrored closely in a Dutch study (Frey *et al.* 2024). The authors examined the weekly reductions in healthcare utilization in 2020 and 2021. In one week of March 2020 there was a decline of 300,000 individuals who should have been admitted to hospital (some for urgent treatment). This reduction varied according to socio-economic status. Individuals living below the poverty line in the Netherlands saw reductions of 6.1 per cent for "medium" urgent procedures, compared with 4.3 per cent for those above the poverty line. The same inequality existed when comparing those with a migrant background and those without. With regard to specific conditions, reductions in very urgent treatment for cancer were almost twice as large for women compared to men, and also much greater for older people. Whether this is due to fewer referrals from primary care (general practitioners) or concerns about hospital attendance is unclear. Nonetheless, delayed cancer screening may have an impact on cancer incidence (and inequalities therein) in years to come.

In the US, Wang *et al.* (2021) noted that some health facilities closed during the pandemic, while people who lost their jobs found themselves without employer health insurance. In particular, "minorities and people with low educational attainment and low incomes have experienced disproportionate job loss and delayed care" (Wang *et al.* 2021: 2). Using mobile phone data, their study in North Carolina revealed that small areas with higher percentages of older people, ethnic minorities and low-income households lacking a car had limited use of healthcare both before and during the pandemic.

Is there other evidence of a geography to these disruptions to care? A report from the UK's Health Foundation in 2020[15] suggests there is, although this tracked waiting lists only until the middle of 2020 so it is very much an interim picture. Nonetheless, while the authors suggest that the pandemic was having a considerable effect on waiting lists in England as a whole, access to elective care was worse in some parts of the country than others. Specifically, with regard to new treatments, the South West had a reduction of 29 per cent compared with 2019, partly because the number of Covid cases and hospitalizations were relatively low; in the North West the percentage reduction was greater (34 per cent).

Elsewhere in the world, household survey data from Latin America and the Caribbean (Herrera *et al.* 2024) revealed that, in both 2020 and 2021, there was a clear social class gradient. There were fewer disruptions among wealthier households, or those in work and reporting less food insecurity. Specifically, about 7.7 per cent of households in the lowest wealth quartile reported disruption to healthcare in 2021, compared with only 2.3 per cent in the top wealth quartile. A broader study across 16 diverse countries (Abel *et al.* 2024) drew from online surveys, comprising just over 22,000 responses. Results suggested that, in low and middle-income countries (including Brazil, Ghana, Uganda,

15. www.health.org.uk/publications/long-reads/elective-care-in-england-assessing-the-impact-of-COVID-19-and-where-next

South Africa and India), there were considerable inequalities in securing appointments in primary care, or getting admitted to hospital. The authors suggest that a wider take-up of digital services (discussed in the Chapter 7) may dilute these inequalities.

Evidence suggests that women's access to healthcare services in general, and to family planning in particular, worsened during the pandemic. In a wide-ranging survey across 76 countries, and drawing on almost 12,500 respondents, Padmaja and Behera (2023) found that women on low incomes and living in rural areas reported worse access to contraceptive services, in part because of the closure of pharmacies and travel restrictions. But this varies according to world region, with those living in African countries reporting the most difficulty in accessing contraception facilities.

Concluding remarks

A picture painted in this chapter can only convey, in the broadest brushstrokes, the suffering caused in zones of conflict by the lack of an adequate assemblage of healthcare: comprising clinical staff, clinical facilities, medicines, and food and water. Powerful actors can ensure that such assemblages are fractured or demolished. This is as true in the DRC as it is in Gaza. The willingness of international aid groups to provide assistance is stymied by such actors, whether armed groups on the ground or, more insidiously, nation states that do all they can to block attempts to come to the rescue of vulnerable populations. Only determined journalists and reporters can begin to tell the distressing stories of those suffering without medical and other assistance in war-torn areas.

In a different context the same constraints on delivering healthcare can arise when armed groups disrupt supply chains during natural disasters. Haiti offered a compelling example, as did Myanmar, both countries affected by earthquakes and both seeing either gangs or armed militia blocking the delivery of aid. In a very different setting, we saw how, in New Orleans, some healthcare workers left the region in the wake of the hurricane.

Last, we considered the impact of disease outbreaks (Ebola) and the Covid-19 pandemic on access to healthcare. In the former case we saw how an already fragile healthcare system in the most affected countries (particularly Sierra Leone) was severely tested by the virus, with some writers (notably Paul Farmer) criticizing the over-emphasis on containment rather than clinical care, while others took an opposing view. The lack of equipment needed to provide care was a common theme.

That theme – be it a lack of personal protective equipment or vaccines – runs through the discussion of Covid-19. We saw that, as the pandemic began to wane in later 2022, well over two-thirds of people across the world had been given a vaccine; but that proportion was only one-quarter in low and middle-income countries. In countries with good health infrastructure for vaccine production and delivery, access to the vaccine was inevitably better. In high-income countries such as the US we noted disparities according to ethnicity and geography, with those living in rural areas finding access to clinics for vaccination more problematic, although whether this is simply due to geographical constraints or vaccine scepticism or hesitancy requires further examination.

Missing from this chapter is a consideration of the care that can and should be given to those seeking new lives in countries of the Global North, whether they are crossing the English Channel to the UK or crossing from Mexico into the US. It is these "mobilities" that are the subject of the next chapter. As we will see, it is less a question of "who cares", but rather "who does not care". To that end, we have seen in this chapter that one group's domination of another means that care is withheld, or actively impeded, whether in Gaza or Myanmar.

Further reading

On Ebola the standard text is Farmer (2020) which, at over 650 pages, is lengthy but superbly written and meticulously documented; as an aside, there is also a brief description of Covid-19.

The journal *Conflict and Health*[16] is a valuable source of material. For up-to-date information on attacks on healthcare workers see the Safeguarding Health in Conflict Coalition website[17] and on the need for better protection of them see Brennan and Sheraz (2024).

On humanitarianism and Covid-19 the paper by Herrick and colleagues (2022) is a must-read. For a good discussion of equity issues regarding Covid-19 vaccination see Santangelo *et al.* (2024) and Rydland *et al.* (2022). There is a growing literature on unequal access to healthcare during the pandemic. Some of the literature cited by Abel *et al.* (2024) provides a useful starting point, but there is no substitute for a proper literature search (for example, using PubMed).

16. https://conflictandhealth.biomedcentral.com
17. https://safeguarding-health.com/

7

MOBILITIES AND ACCESS TO HEALTHCARE

> Demagogues and national security experts now look askance at many of those who move, defining mobility as dangerous and threatening, while immobility is seen as normal and necessary for political and personal security.
>
> Glick Schiller and Salazar (2013: 184)

In two previous books I have examined the links between migration and health (Gatrell 2011: chs 6–7) and the health of those being displaced from their homes in search of a better, safer life (Gatrell 2023: ch. 5). Neither of those books gave sufficient attention to associations between movement and *access to healthcare*, and this chapter seeks to fill that gap.

In a book that is concerned with the geographies of unequal access to healthcare the question of how and where people move – either daily, or more long term – to seek out such care is clearly central. In the most obvious sense people travel to a local health centre or a local or regional hospital, and depending on their circumstances this might be relatively straightforward or very demanding. To take another obvious example, people might wait for healthcare to come to them, as when an ambulance or emergency vehicle is required to attend an accident (see Wendy's story in the introductory chapter). In all these cases there are social dimensions and inequalities, not least in the costs of travel but also the costs to health of waiting. There are also issues involving the technologies brought to bear in healthcare and whether some of these negate the need to move; instead, the care may be delivered remotely. Yet this is never merely a technical exercise as it raises issues of whether or not the technologies are acceptable to, or help, the recipient, as well as whether some people and groups have better access to such technologies than do others.

Then again, as we saw in the introduction, those delivering healthcare are invariably mobile; they have to get to work, or get to their clients and patients. Some, like nurse Sadia Khan (Chapter 1), may face considerable challenges getting to work. In other contexts, healthcare professionals move from one country to another to seek better employment. As we see later, they may not always find themselves welcome. For some people, crossing international borders is relatively straightforward; for others, the border is a rigid barrier obstructing movement and using an assemblage of tools designed to keep people out.

Welcome is not always extended to mobile marginalized populations, such as Gypsy, Roma and Traveller people, and the healthcare of these communities needs attention (Box 7.1). So too do the needs of those fleeing zones of conflict or resource depletion in order to find safer homes. Whether or not they are able to access healthcare in the countries they find themselves in is also a theme considered here. There is a clear contrast with those who have the means to seek out medical treatments (surgery, or dental care, for example) overseas; so-called "medical (or health) tourism" is also considered in this chapter. So too is the application of mobile devices and related technologies to healthcare and we consider whether, how and for whom it improves patients' access to treatment.

BOX 7.1 MOBILE COMMUNITIES: GYPSY, ROMA AND TRAVELLERS

A popular view of mobile communities living in the Global North is to lump them all together as "Gypsies" (a label that some accept and others find offensive) but it is more appropriate to refer to Gypsy, Roma and Travellers (GRT), acknowledging that there is a risk of conflating groups with different cultural backgrounds, and conceivably differing healthcare wants and needs. The commonalities are nomadism and a strong sense of family.

There are various factors impeding access to healthcare among these communities, the members of which have to contend with being stigmatized and discriminated racially. Aside from these structural barriers some members of the groups may have poor literacy and limited knowledge of how to engage with statutory healthcare systems as well as possible distrust of these bodies. Safarian and colleagues (2024) have explored these issues in some detail, drawing on interviews with Bulgarian Roma people living in London and Leicester and with the research team that includes Roma people. Healthcare was provided less by formal primary care teams (in GP surgeries) and more by family members. One interviewee said: "We have a GP in the UK, but we do not go to the doctor, it takes too long to arrange an interpreter; we treat ourselves with medicines from Bulgaria. We also share medicines with others who need them" (in Safarian *et al.* 2024: 3). Some people returned to Bulgaria to obtain medical care.

There are several reviews of research on access to healthcare for GRT groups (e.g. McFadden *et al.* 2018) but a relative lack of detailed empirical studies.

First, however, I want to explain why I refer to "mobilities" in the chapter heading.

The mobilities turn in social science

The term "mobilities" was first popularized by the late John Urry who sees it as a "broader project of establishing a movement-driven social science" (Urry 2007: 18). Such movement includes not only the people and objects "doing" the move, but also the physical and material infrastructure that enables (or impedes) it. To this, we can add people enabling or impeding human movement, and, in this chapter those enabling or impeding healthcare delivery. There are, therefore, assemblages or networks of people and things that are the focus of mobilities research.

As noted elsewhere (Gatrell 2023) early mobilities research focused attention on the "kinetic elite", those well-heeled, well-travelled passengers whose experience of, for example, the airport contrasted with those enabling such travel: the baggage handlers and ground staff and others who were distinctly immobile, such as those using the airport as a place of refuge. I think it fair to say too that early mobilities researchers gave more attention to those moving around the Global North rather than the Global South. For example, Tim Cresswell's ground-breaking book (2006) was subtitled: *Mobility in the Modern Western World*. In a healthcare context this is reflected in the academic interest in "health tourism". Although that literature has developed independently of the mobilities turn it too has focused much of its attention on those who can afford to travel from countries in the Global North to those in the Global South. This is considered later.

More recently Mimi Sheller (2018) has written on mobility justice (Box 7.2) and, as we will see in the next section, this is clearly relevant when considering access to healthcare for those desperate for a new home.

BOX 7.2 MOBILITY JUSTICE

For Sheller (2018) mobility justice refers to a set of rights that should be afforded to people's movements and she illustrates these at various scales, from the body, street, city, nation-state and planet. Taking these in turn we can consider how individual bodies (most obviously, those that are physically impaired) might be impeded from moving around and this is seen when navigating streets and cities that make some movement challenging. At the national scale there are, as we see in this chapter, constraints at borders, involving those people, materials and infrastructure that inhibit cross-border movement. At the planetary scale we see movements that are triggered by climate change and political conflict. Sheller sets out "rights" that should apply at each of these scales. Some examples are:

- there should be no trampling, endangering, or depriving others of their capability for mobility;
- public systems of transport shall not arbitrarily deny access to some groups because of physical barriers;

- there should be a right to refuge for those fleeing violence, persecution, and loss of domicile by war;
- people displaced by climate change shall have a right to resettlement in other countries, especially in those countries that contributed most to climate change.

Clearly, some of these rights, notably the last one, are subject to considerable public debate and, in many cases, anger and violent opposition.

Sheller suggests that mobility justice provides a vehicle for illustrating that power and inequality inform and control movement of people and resources. Such movements are laden with unevenness and inequity.

Healthcare access for refugees and asylum seekers

"People move. Healthcare facilities stay in place" (Follis *et al.* 2025: 2). In their important collection, Follis and colleagues examine the constraints faced by refugees, asylum seekers and temporary workers in seeking to access health services; although as we see later, healthcare facilities do not always "stay in place". "In many countries, they face structural and infrastructural barriers to medical care in national health systems typically designed to serve sedentary populations (i.e. domestically settled)" (Follis *et al.* 2025: 2). There are other barriers of course, aided by the rhetoric of politicians for whom immigration is something of a dirty word. In this section I consider access for people who are displaced and seek healthcare in another country, having dealt in Chapter 6 with the issues of access for those displaced *internally* during periods of crisis and conflict.

The US/Mexico border is one of the most high-profile regions of immigration, acting as a point of entry into the US by those coming from Guatemala, El Salvador and Honduras, as well as Mexico. More recently, source countries have included Venezuela and Nicaragua. The US Customs and Border Protection (CBP) processes migrants and asylum seekers when they arrive at the border. Such "processing" might simply involve deporting people. Those seeking asylum are screened if there is a "credible fear" if they return to their country; if eligible they are released but must attend an immigration court.

The erection and heightening of the border wall first introduced by President Trump in 2017 has had serious consequences for those desperate enough to try scaling it. The number of traumatic injuries and deaths has been documented by Tenorio *et al.* (2024) but the relevance to this book is the significant increase in hospital admissions and therefore the pressure on the healthcare system. For example, in El Paso (Texas) while there were no admissions due to border falls in 2016 there were almost 20 each month in 2021. Most of these injured people are simply discharged after treatment, with no follow-up, or they are returned to CBP custody.

So-called "qualified aliens" (including refugees and those seeking asylum) are permitted to access healthcare, including Medicaid, but this is denied to "undocumented migrants" (unless there is a medical emergency). The latter have to rely on a safety net that includes some not-for-profit hospitals, and community and migrant health centres. Thus there is a contrast between the treatment of asylum seekers and that of undocumented arrivals.

The publicity given to migration at the US/Mexico border overshadows other refugee flows in Central and South America, notably those from Venezuela (mostly to Colombia, but many seeking to reach the US), in what has been described as "the largest displacement crisis in the world, with almost 7.7 million migrants and refugees as of August 2023".[1] The irregular nature of this migration (and hence, lack of insurance) means poor access to healthcare, a feature shared by those displaced internally because of armed conflict in Colombia. The Colombian government set up the Permiso Especial de Permanencia (PEP) scheme that provides temporary access to education, work and healthcare for Venezuelan migrants. But barriers to healthcare remain, of which the three main ones are a lack of documentation, distance to health centres and poor access to transport (Diaz *et al.* 2023). The same authors report that some Venezuelans are turned away from health centres because of xenophobia. The community health workers interviewed by Diaz and colleagues suggested that mobile health teams could help improve access (see below, pp. 150–3).

People seeking asylum in the UK are entitled to the same NHS care as the settled population. However, while there may be entitlement (*potential access*) the number of barriers (bureaucratic, organizational, logistical) placed in their path means that *realized access* is a different matter. As Follis *et al.* (2025: 5) put it: "In a healthcare system already beset by the challenges of austerity and scarcity, sedentary bias additionally accounts for the limited capability to follow the movements of these patients and their health data". This is revealed very clearly in Lonergan's study of the experiences of vulnerable pregnant migrants in Britain (see Follis *et al.* 2025). Official NHS guidance is for "continuity of care" but this rings hollow for those who see little or no "reproductive justice". As one adviser from the voluntary sector puts it:

> *what happens is that women who are pregnant, despite there being a policy around this, are moved around the Home Office estate, if you like, and can be moved at very short-notice. And the impact that has on their antenatal care can be really serious. There's no continuity of care built into the system. So it causes a lot of problems for women who are put into, you know, moved from one hotel to another, to a hostel, then moved again* (in Follis *et al.* 2025: 114–15).

1. www.csis.org/analysis/persistence-venezuelan-migrant-and-refugee-crisis

For some healthcare workers there are professional and moral dilemmas in dealing with undocumented arrivals at international borders. These dilemmas have been explored by Lafaut (2021) in his study of access to healthcare in Belgium based on interviews with 45 healthcare workers. He reveals that some of these do not enquire about residency status: as he puts it, they are "purposefully inattentive" (Lafaut 2021: 1). Such dilemmas are also explored in a British context by Potter and Meier (see Follis *et al.* 2025: 29) who suggest that healthcare professionals engage in "emotional borderwork" where they try to "negotiate the dilemmas presented by the duty to put patients first on the one hand, and the formal requirements of the hostile environment on the other".

There are other stories of marginalized people struggling to navigate healthcare systems in a foreign country. Escriva and colleagues (see Follis *et al.* 2025) tell us about a Moroccan fruit-picker worker in Spain, diagnosed with cancer but left badly neglected. Her case is symptomatic of "the afflictions and illnesses of marginalized individuals [that] accumulate as they migrate annually through agricultural circuits spanning international borders. Neither employers nor public services are sufficiently prepared to offer protection and pauses for healing within this system of intensive farming" (Follis *et al.* 2025: 63).

In all these cases we read of the importance of "non-governmental, voluntary and other third-sector organizations", since statutory services are poorly prepared to offer assistance. In addition, there are activist groups providing information and support. One such, in England, is Patients Not Passports, which is "organising to end racist immigration controls in the NHS".[2]

Moving health professionals

Connell and Walton-Roberts (2016) have, quite correctly, noted that health geographers' concerns with access to healthcare have tended to ignore the labour of those employed in such services. In a book with a main title *Who Cares?* it is essential to look at the geographies of the skilled healthcare workforce and, in this section, to examine the impact of their migration on the places they have come from and the places they now work. I have examined some of these issues in an earlier book (Gatrell 2011: 169–74), while Connell and Walton-Roberts (2016) explore these issues in detail, speaking of the "deterritorialization" of healthcare and observing (with a nod to "assemblages"; see above, pp. 27–8) that "patients, workers (and pharmaceuticals and scans) move considerable distances" (Connell & Walton-Roberts 2016: 163).

The movement of health professionals can take several forms. It can include the movement of workers from the public sector to the private sector, internal migration, and migration from one country to another. Sixty years ago there were major worries

2. See https://patientsnotpassports.co.uk/

Table 7.1 Emigration rate to OECD countries for medical workforce from countries of origin (2015–16)

Country	*Emigration rate (%)*
St Lucia	97
Sao Tome & Principe	82
Liberia	76
St Vincent & the Grenadines	75
Dominica	70
Samoa	64
Zimbabwe	64
Malawi	58
Antigua & Barbuda	57
Somalia	57
Sierra Leone	54
Guyana	53

Note: The emigration rate is expressed as a percentage of the total working in the country.
Source: Socha-Dietrich and Dumont (2021).

about the so-called "brain drain" from well-resourced countries such as the UK to other countries (notably, Australia). The main focus here is on movement from countries in the Global South to countries in the Global North, but there are of course other regional flows. We need to assess the consequences such migration has for the health systems in Global South countries, and the mechanisms in place to ensure this is ethical. We next consider the "value" (or otherwise) placed on skilled workers moving from the Global South to the Global North.

In 2010 the World Health Organization (WHO) established a "Global Code of Practice on the International Recruitment of Health Personnel", that sought to address issues of workforce retention in countries of the Global South. It "provides ethical principles applicable to the international recruitment of health personnel in a manner that strengthens the health systems of developing countries, countries with economies in transition and small island states".[3] In 2022 its report suggested that 15 per cent of skilled healthcare workers were employed in countries other than their country of birth or where they first qualified (Kamarulzaman *et al.* 2022). The volume of this movement seems to be increasing. For example, the number of doctors emigrating from India and Pakistan in 1990 was 46,000 and 7,752 respectively, but in 2014 this had risen to 88,000 and 26,500 (Kamarulzaman *et al.* 2022). Table 7.1 shows countries where over 50 per cent of the total medical workforce emigrated to Organisation for Economic Co-operation and Development (OECD) countries in 2015–16. African and (small) Caribbean countries figure prominently. More doctors born in those countries are working in OECD countries other than their birthplace.

3. www.who.int/publications/i/item/wha68.32

There are both push and pull factors at work, including poor working conditions, low salaries and political disruption, with the attractions of better conditions and remuneration and a safer political environment. But there are, inevitably, equity consequences for the "sender" countries as these movements denude health systems and populations of expertise and, if there is insufficient local skilled workforce, the public's health will suffer.

The WHO Code is a voluntary one. Tankwanchi *et al.* (2015) have monitored the adoption of the Code with reference to the migration of doctors from sub-Saharan countries to the US. They note that, in 2013, there were just under 12,000 such doctors working in the US – mostly in the large cities and representing about 1.3 per cent of the medical workforce. However, about 16 per cent of these entered the US after the Code of Practice (CoP) was established, suggesting it might have relatively little "teeth". The authors put it starkly: "Although unanimously ratified by all WHO member states, the non-binding nature of the CoP reflects an all-too-rhetorical and reactionary policy, preserving the interests of doctor-receiving countries while denying any serious leverage to source countries that lose their health personnel" (Tankwanchi *et al.* 2015: 10).

The UK Government revised its own code in 2021, aiming to ensure that recruitment is ethical and transparent and will "protect and promote health and social care system sustainability through international co-operation by ensuring safeguards and support for countries with the most pressing health and social care workforce challenges".[4] There is a long "red list" of countries from which active recruitment is not permitted; this includes all sub-Saharan countries as well as Afghanistan, Bangladesh, Pakistan and Pacific island states. Despite this, the UK's NHS recruitment of doctors from overseas continues to increase, notably from countries in the Global South. Eaton *et al.* (2023) report that in 2022, out of a total of about 357,000 registered doctors 147,000 of them trained outside the UK and of those 79,000 received their training in the 57 poorest countries in the world. The same authors note the inverse relationship between doctors per head of population in low and middle-income countries and indicators such as maternal and infant mortality rates in those countries. They suggest that the UK Government's revised code of practice for international recruitment "is blatantly not being followed" (Eaton *et al.* 2023: 256). The same issue applies to nursing staff, with a post-Brexit "surge" in the number being recruited from red list countries. Two-thirds (just under 47,000) of all nurses in the UK who started working there between 2021 and 2024 were trained outside the UK or Europe. As the minister in charge of health and social care (Wes Streeting) noted, this is "immoral".[5]

4. www.gov.uk/government/publications/code-of-practice-for-the-international-recruitment-of-health-and-social-care-personnel/code-of-practice-for-the-international-recruitment-of-health-and-social-care-personnel-in-england
5. https://www.theguardian.com/society/2025/mar/21/post-brexit-reliance-on-nhs-staff-from-red-list-countries-is-unethical-streeting-says

The consequences for "sender" countries are profound, leading inevitably to weakening of health services provision. In a telling phrase Connell and Walton-Roberts (2016) refer to this as a "service vacuum" and stress that this gap refers not only to medical staff but to other skilled health workers as well – notably, nurses, the great majority of whom are women. Despite suggestions that those arriving to work in the UK (and elsewhere) remit parts of their salaries back "home" these cannot compensate for the loss of skilled staff and there is little evidence that skills acquired in destination countries are transferred back to the origin countries. While such migration helps to improve access to healthcare in wealthier countries it weakens access in sender countries. There are inequities therefore in relative provision and consequently moral and ethical issues. Exploring these issues Mpofu *et al.* (2016) argue that we should devote less attention to the needs of such wealthy countries and that instead such countries should be guided by principles of justice that consider the needs of health systems on a global scale. Otherwise, the (human) rights of those living in Global South countries are being ignored.

What of the consequences of these Global South–Global North flows for "destination" countries and, in particular, the challenges faced by healthcare workers moving to them? There is an anti-immigration mindset in many countries of the Global North. Beresford and Sodero (2025) suggest that, in the UK, the NHS is "being absorbed into a wider anti-immigration agenda", a mindset that appears to be adopted in government circles with the UK's Secretary of State for Health and Social Care, Wes Streeting, arguing that the country needs to be "self-sufficient in terms of building, training, and drawing on our own homegrown talent".[6] This is at odds with the NHS Confederation which counters that "immigration is of net benefit to the NHS and an incoming government should explore ways to make international recruitment to the sector as easy as possible, alongside efforts to grow the domestic workforce".[7] Regardless, there is evidence that racism and anti-migrant rhetoric – as instanced by abuse directed at doctors who trained overseas – is driving them out of the UK. Almost 5,000 doctors who qualified in another country left the UK in 2024, an increase of 26 per cent from the previous year.[8]

If these are contrasting views at the national level how does an "anti-immigration agenda" translate into the real experiences of those working in the health service? An important paper (Allan *et al.* 2004) excavated some of these experiences drawing on focus groups comprising 67 internationally recruited nurses working in three British cities. One Nigerian nurse said: "*No matter if they know you are an overseas qualified nurse, the way you are being approached or addressed is quite different completely from the so-called UK-trained nurses because they look at you as if you don't have anything upstairs at all*" (quoted in Allan *et al.* 2004). The authors suggest that their findings are

6. https://inews.co.uk/news/politics/over-reliance-migration-nhs-wes-streeting-3063238
7. www.nhsconfed.org/articles/immigration-harming-nhs
8. https://www.theguardian.com/society/2025/nov/21/overseas-trained-doctors-leaving-uk-record-numbers

indicative of institutional racism in the health service. Generalizing this we can argue that nurses (and doctors) may be stigmatized or "othered" because of their skin colour; they are subject to a form of "symbolic violence", a form of suffering because of being devalued or lacking recognition by others. This is confirmed in research by Alexis *et al.* (2006) with a smaller sample of Black and minority ethnic nurses coming to England. The main finding here was a lack of equal opportunities as the following extract makes clear:

> *Opportunities are not given to us equally as I have been on this ward for three years. Promised by my manager that the next available vacancy, I should apply. Went for the job and it was given to someone far junior to me. Another vacancy came up and I was unsuccessful. I just could not understand what I had done wrong on both occasions. I just can't help but think that I was denied this promotion because I am an overseas nurse and promotion is blighted because of my colour of my skin.* (quoted in Alexis *et al.* 2006: 133)

Sowemimo (2023: 233–40) explores these issues in a compelling way, based on her personal experiences, and noting (235) "ill-informed, racist stereotypes that surround health professionals from overseas".

Mobile health teams

This section considers the ways in which clinical teams can provide mobile care rather than delivering it in fixed locations – hospital and clinics. This builds on the previous chapter which considered the provision of care in emergency contexts, whether these be conflict zones or natural disasters. Here, my concern is less with "acute" delivery and more the everyday delivery of, and access to, healthcare on the move.

Yu *et al.* (2017: 1) suggest that mobile health clinics (MHCs) are "an innovative model of healthcare delivery that could help alleviate health disparities in vulnerable populations and individuals with chronic diseases". The authors' discussion predates the Covid-19 pandemic and many of those reading this book will have experienced mobile vaccination clinics (for a good example see the analysis of the "Vaccine on Wheels" initiative in India; Patel *et al.* 2024). The present discussion asks whether such clinics address the needs of underserved communities, improving access that might otherwise not be obtained.

Evidence from the operation of MHCs in the US certainly suggests they improve access to potentially vulnerable groups. Updating the earlier description by Yu and colleagues Malone *et al.* (2020) draw on a database of about 2,000 MHCs, and a survey of some of these reveals that over half the clinics target uninsured, low income populations, with just over one-third of the clinics serving homeless persons and rural communities. People of colour are over-represented in the sample of users. For example, while the 2010 Census reported 13 per cent of the population as Black American the percentage of that population using the clinics was 35 per cent. The focus of MHC work is on primary care and preventative services (including screening). The authors estimate that up to 7 million visits are paid each year to these clinics.

Mobile clinics in principle offer a means of overcoming the transport difficulties of getting to appointments (although they also require patients to be in the right place at the right time) and can circumvent lengthy waiting times for appointments. They work in, and for neighbourhood communities, providing potential links between health and social care services and potentially addressing the social determinants of health. A good example of the latter is the Outreach Van Project (OVP), created in 2007 by students at Boston University's School of Medicine.[9] This serves a mainly Hispanic community in East Boston, where one-fifth of the population lives below the poverty line. About half of OVP's clients are immigrants from Central America who do not speak English and therefore need help in being directed to primary care and welfare services.

Rabiou and colleagues (2024) have explored the use of mobile health teams in south-east Niger, close to the Nigerian border, a region affected by both armed conflict and flooding and one where only half the population is within 5 kilometres of a health clinic. Travel difficulties are exacerbated during the wet season. These mobile teams provide immunization and antenatal care, along with advice about family planning, reaching over 42,000 people during a three-month period. Such clinics offer invaluable healthcare elsewhere in West Africa as well as in challenging environments in countries such as Haiti. Yet there are practical difficulties, not least letting target populations know when and where the teams will call.

Mobile health clinics have a particular value in serving Indigenous communities. In Queensland, Australia, for example, a "Mobile Outreach Boomerang" (MOB) van (Figure 7.1) serves Aboriginal and Torres Strait Islander peoples, providing access to primary healthcare (including to primary and secondary school students) in a culturally appropriate way (Askew *et al.* 2023). These findings are generalized in a review of MHCs that serve Indigenous populations in Canada, the US and New Zealand, as well as Australia (Beks *et al.* 2020). This paper maps the locations of such clinics in Australia and Canada, revealing their distribution in the more remote areas. As in the US, most clinics are funded by a mix of government and philanthropic sources.

Care must be taken not to exaggerate the benefits of such clinics. While they may well improve geographic access for hard-to-reach communities, some studies draw attention to other issues that only emerge when users are spoken to. A good example is the study of clinics in KwaZulu-Natal, South Africa (Nkosi 2023). While the convenience of access is a benefit ("respondents highlighted that the mobile clinic brings health care to their doorsteps"; Nkosi 2023: 4), there were complaints about lack of privacy during consultations and limitations on what services (and medical staff) were provided. As one female respondent put it: "*The nurses do give out medication if they*

9. www.bumc.bu.edu/camed/student-affairs/student-life/service-learning/outreach-van-project-2/

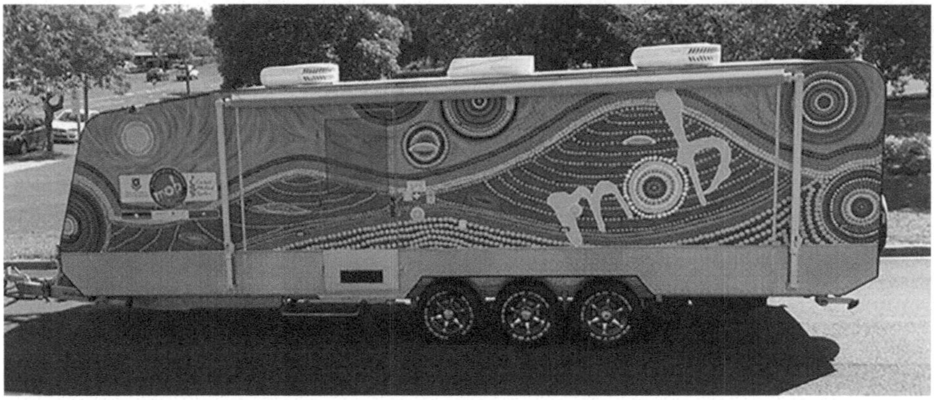

Figure 7.1 The Mobile Outreach Boomerang (MOB) van in Queensland, Australia
Source: Courtesy of Daryl Tan, New South Wales Government, Australia.

have enough on that day but the issue of lack of medication is happening more regularly now than before" (Nkosi 2023: 4). Similar issues are reported in a study of mobile clinics established by Médecins Sans Frontières in the Somali region of Ethiopia (Sahelie *et al.* 2025). This study of a pastoralist community revealed that distance to clinic sites was a barrier to access, with average journey times on foot taking over 100 minutes. In general, the limited opening hours of the clinics, coupled with large numbers of patients and problems in referring them for further treatment, created difficulties in accessing healthcare.

Some mobile services are delivered on water, not land. Garnelo and colleagues (2020) have explored the distinctive nature of healthcare provision for Indigenous riverside peoples living in Amazonia. This is based on establishing "Fluvial Family Health Teams" that operate in fluvial mobile units (FMUs) that may take 12 hours to travel from Manaus, the state capital of Amazonas (Figure 7.2). An FMU is staffed by doctors, nurses, dentists and pharmacists, as well as boat crew, and carries facilities for consultations, dental care, vaccinations and laboratory analysis. The authors conducted interviews with both service users (living in 38 settlements along the banks of the Negro River) and members of the FMUs providing primary care in this part of the State. Their research paints a rich and vivid picture of how care is delivered. Clearly, only basic primary care can be provided and those accessing the FMU still incur costs in travelling to the unit or getting to hospital for more specialized care. Further, the health professionals only "have limited knowledge of the way of life of the rural populations under their responsibility" (Garnelo *et al.* 2020: 9) and rely on local community health workers for enabling better connections to the local populations. Nonetheless, the quality of antenatal care (for example) provided by the FMU is little different from that offered in urban primary care facilities.

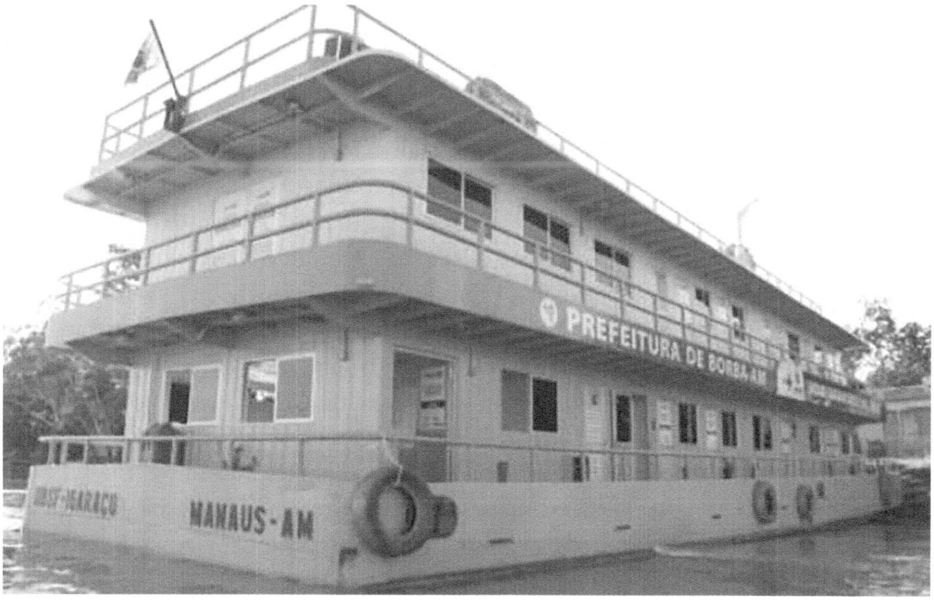

Figure 7.2 A fluvial mobile clinic in Amazonas state, Brazil
Source: International Journal of Nursing and Midwifery: doi: 10.5897/IJNM2017.0256.

In Peru, the *Amazon Hope* river ship, operated by the charity Vine Trust, serves those living in the Loreto region of Peru (Limaye *et al.* 2018). The region is sparsely populated, with over half living below the official poverty level, and the ship provides preventative, medical and dental care to over 160 remote communities, with visits every three months. Survey research by Limaye *et al.* (2018) reveals that the *Amazon Hope* "is able to reach a population in extreme poverty with multiple determinants of poor health, including limited access to reproductive health services" (11). However, for some survey respondents, better notification of the ship's visits was needed and while the ship improved service access for vulnerable people there was a significant under-representation of young men.

In Africa, Partners in Health[10] document the replacement of an ageing canoe on the Hoffman River in Liberia with motorized transport to provide access to a hospital. The town chief acknowledged that "*This means a lot to us. Our pregnant women and mothers will use it to go for their vaccines and other health services; and farmers will use it to transport their produce to markets*".

10. www.pih.org/article/modern-canoe-gives-remote-community-access-health-care

Moving for care

In Gatrell (2011: 174–8) I discussed medical or health "tourism", where people travel overseas to seek healthcare that may be unavailable or overly expensive at home. Such travel might be from one country in the Global North to another but recent interest has been in travel from countries in the Global North to those in the Global South (notably, but not exclusively, India and Thailand). Rather than rehearsing the considerable literature on this topic (see Brown *et al.* 2018: ch. 13 for an overview) my focus here is on the equity issues, with particular attention to how and whether such "tourism" has any impacts on the health services in those countries being visited. There are frequently articles in the popular press that recount "horror stories" about botched dental or cosmetic care consumed overseas but such penalties of accessing poor care are not considered here. Brown *et al.* (2018: 234) observe that some in the popular press refer to alternative "horror stories" about "overseas migrants flocking to the [UK] to make use of free access to health care services". Further, while some might criticize the words medical/health "tourist" as an unfortunate descriptor of someone seeking urgent or much-needed care overseas, others (notably Smith 2012) consider it quite appropriate given how private hospitals overseas market the hotel-like experience for such consumers.

As Snyder and Crooks (2012) noted, the demand for treatment by those prepared to pay to access healthcare in the Global South may lead to poorer access for domestic populations if it means that resources that would otherwise accrue to them are diverted to support private clinics treating overseas clients. Such resources might include those better devoted to primary care rather than high-tech acute care in private hospitals. Ramirez de Arellano (2007) illustrates some of these issues with reference to the Bumrungrad *International* Hospital (note the italics) in Bangkok, Thailand (Figure 7.3). The hospital's website says the following: "Bumrungrad is an internationally accredited, multi-specialty hospital listed on the Stock Exchange of Thailand since 1989. One of the largest private hospitals in Southeast Asia, Bumrungrad International Hospital cares for over 1.1 million patients from more than 190 countries annually".[11] As Figure 7.3 suggests, it bears all the hallmarks of a plush hotel, not unlike Auckland's Ascot Hospital described in Chapter 2 (pp. 9–10).

Although the precise details may now be dated, Ramirez de Arellano asserts that "the fact that the private health sector in Bangkok has more gamma knife, computed tomography (CT) scan, and mammography capacity than England is evidence of the distortions that occur" (Ramirez de Arellano 2007: 196). She refers to hospitals such as Bumrungrad as "islands of medical excellence in a sea of medical neglect". Connell (2011: 263) refers to the "internal brain drain" in the country as clinicians move from the periphery to the

11. https://www.bumrungrad.com/en/about-us/bumrungrad-international-hospital

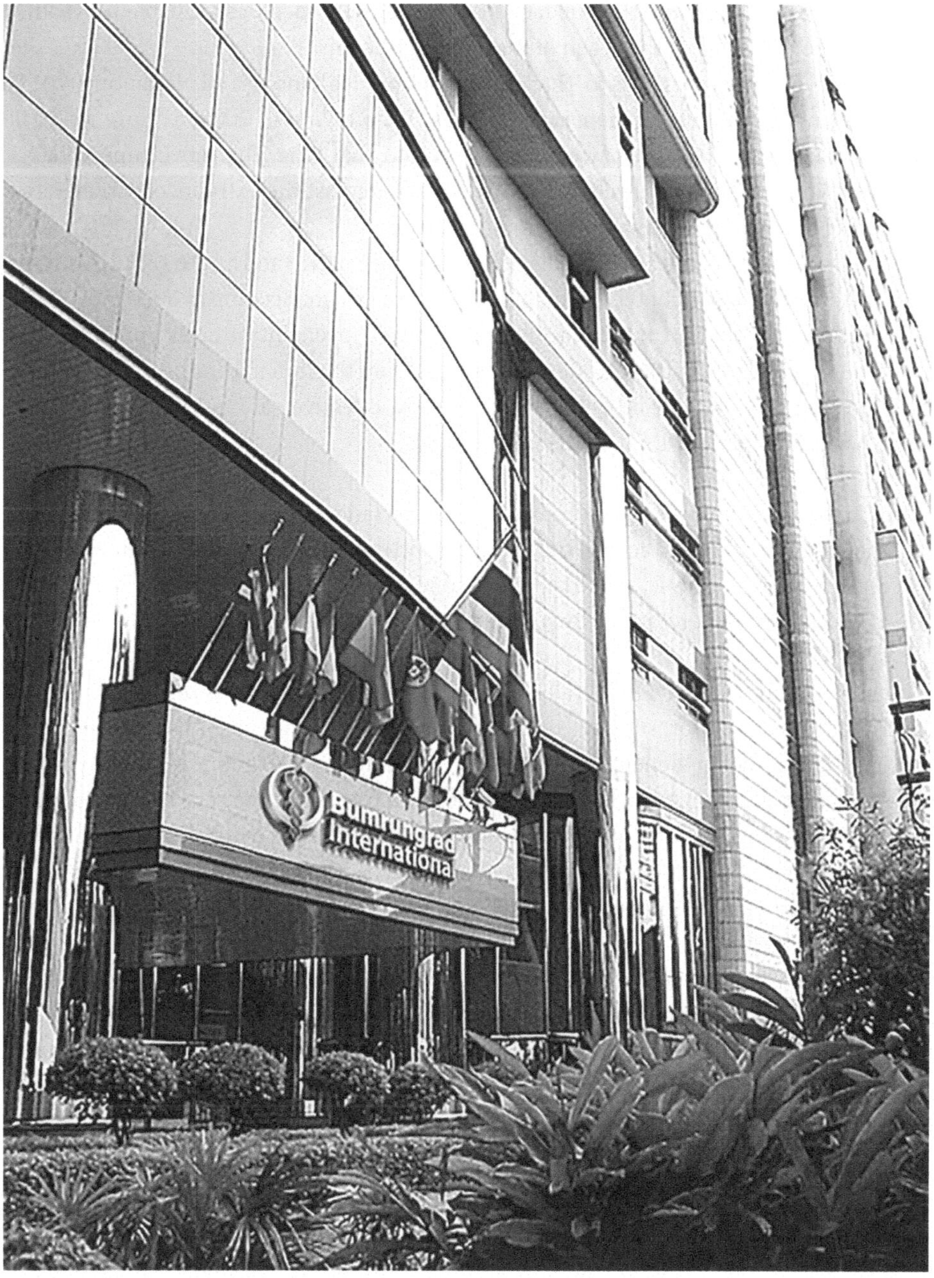

Figure 7.3 The Bumrungrad International Hospital, Bangkok, Thailand
Source: Wikipedia.

centre (Bangkok). He also notes the fact that the excellent facilities available to wealthy "tourists" are well beyond the reach of most Thai nationals.

There are, of course, benefits to Thailand's economy. NaRanong and NaRanong (2011) suggest that medical tourism generated about US$1.5 billion in 2008, a figure that will have increased considerably since. But they argue that "the Thai government has a responsibility to balance the welfare of Thai citizens against the extra income generated by medical tourism" (NaRanong & NaRanong 2011: 342).

Similar concerns have arisen in India where Meghani (2013) and Smith (2012) both see medical tourism as an archetypal neoliberal initiative. Meghani compares the movement of potential patients from the UK to India with the movement of health professionals from poorer countries to the UK. Representatives from the Indian healthcare sector visit the UK to market private healthcare in India as a cost-effective, safe and timely alternative to the NHS. Meghani (2013: 792) asks:

> as India cannot provide even basic healthcare (and other necessities such as adequate nutrition and access to clean water and sanitation facilities) to hundreds of millions of its people, should it be subsidizing the cost of treatment for paying patients from richer nations by supporting medical tourism?

Her answer is quite clear: neoliberalism (of which medical tourism is but one facet) has hardly benefited the poorest people in India. However, she does acknowledge that there are some "trickle-down" benefits. One large private sector organization (Apollo Hospitals, working with Samsung) provides mobile clinics that travel to more remote rural regions in India to offer medical care at zero or modest cost. But, as the author concludes, this is "a miniscule fraction of India's poor" (Meghani 2013: 796). Smith (2012) develops these arguments further. She refers to the binary nature of healthcare in India. One is the "high quality and high-priced sector catering to foreigners and affluent nationals", the other being a "resource-constrained and lower-quality sector catering to the majority of the local population" (Smith 2012: 5). Much the same argument is made by Bahri (2024: 2) who comments that "private hospitals thrive on the globalised Indian, high net worth individuals, and medical tourists are just the cherry on top, while poorer people struggle to access healthcare". Clearly, there are issues of human rights and equity to be addressed.

Not all healthcare-seeking is from rich to middle-income countries. Some mobilities are between neighbouring countries in the Global South rather than the long distances involved in some of the movement from those in richer countries to low and middle-income destinations. Ormond and Sulianti (2014), like others, have bemoaned the emphasis on North–South health "tourism", referring to a "Northern bias" and preferring to speak of medical "travel" rather than "tourism". As they note, most medical travel to Thailand is within Southeast Asia. The authors explore the motivations and experiences of Indonesians seeking healthcare in Malaysia, where private hospitals have sought to attract Indonesian patients (to the extent that, by 2007, 80 per cent of international travellers to Malaysia were from Indonesia). Interviews with 35 actors in the system (administrators, travel agents, doctors and travellers) consider the motivations of travellers and how such travel is enabled and undertaken. Some praise the quality of Indonesian treatment. One patient said:

> *Doctors here [in Kuching, Indonesia] are more open, honest, and explain to us whether illnesses can be cured or not. They will keep us informed – giving us the percentage of likelihood for a cure, giving us all the information we need. They are clearer and more open – friendlier, more familiar. Our local doctors ... sometimes hide the truth from us.*

Cost considerations are less important than geographic proximity and cultural similarity, social support networks and confidence in the quality of care and treatment.

In a different region, Bojorquez and colleagues (2024) explore exchanges at the Mexico-Guatemala border, drawing on a large sample of about 4,700 people and almost 75,000 border crossings between March and April 2023. Interviews were conducted with 14 users and service providers. The main reasons for health-related border crossings were to purchase medicines (somewhat cheaper in Mexico, often purchased while crossing for other reasons) but also for maternity and dental care, as well as specialized care (for example, ophthalmology).

The wide-ranging review of literature conducted by Durham and Blondell (2017) suggests that such flows are explained by a lack of services (or their unacceptability) in the home country, with decision-making dependent in part on individual social networks. As well as using social capital people draw on stocks of economic and cultural capital, as Bourdieu (above, pp. 27–8) would suggest. For example, "patients travelling from Indonesia to Malaysia, from Bangladesh to India, or from Yemen to Jordan shared similar languages and cultures" (Durham & Blondell 2017: 9). Similarly, in Thailand the authors report that public hospitals are required to treat patients from neighbouring Myanmar, Lao PDR, Cambodia and Malaysia, "regardless of their financial means" (10). Echoing Bourdieu, the authors conclude that "decisions about investments in healthcare services abroad are structured by social networks, the positions individuals hold within these structures, and their access to other capitals" (11). From a more structuralist perspective we can suggest that medical/health tourism is part of the global health economy, characterized by private profit and the treatment of healthcare as a commodity.

Remote sensing: healthcare at a distance

I borrow the sub-heading here from my earlier book (Gatrell 2011: 178–84). Geography students (and those in allied disciplines) explore remote sensing (usually using satellites) as a set of tools for earth observation monitoring. Here, I appropriate the term to describe how health can be sensed, and care provided, remotely; meaning there is no requirement for a patient and clinician to be co-present. Related literature covers the topic of "m-Health" (mobile health), which embraces a range of digital technologies (including text messaging, social media, apps and so on) to monitor and promote health. However, the focus here is more on the use of "telemedicine" for particular clinical specialties and how accompanying "telehealthcare" can provide supportive care. Here, as elsewhere in this chapter, my primary concern is to examine critically the availability of such technologies and whether any population groups are relatively excluded from accessing them. In a book on the unequal geographies of healthcare, the availability of digital health ought to mean that the relative location of clinician and patient is wholly irrelevant. Nonetheless, while geographic access might indeed be a non-issue there are still questions about other forms of access that are worth considering.

There are many authors and agencies who promote and celebrate the use and benefits of digital health technologies. Such benefits (potential rather than necessarily realized) include putting the client/patient at the centre of their healthcare, giving them better access to health information, personal health records, and greater involvement in monitoring their health without the need for face-to-face consultations. One group of authors (quoted in Hendl & Shukla 2024: 295) assert that: "Unimpeded by geographical boundaries, smartphone-linked wearable sensors, point-of-need diagnostic devices, and medical-grade imaging, all built around real-time data streams and supported by automated clinical decision–support tools, will enable care and enhance our understanding of physiological variability". While such claims are invariably exaggerated there are plenty of examples to illustrate what is possible.

In some parts of England there are "virtual wards", meaning that patient health (for example, blood pressure) can be monitored remotely without the need for hospital appointments (and associated travel and waiting time). Harold Chugg in Devon, England was a beneficiary: "Armed with a computer tablet, a Bluetooth-enabled blood pressure cuff and weighing scales, Harold returned to his farm near Chulmleigh in north Devon and logged his own symptoms and measurements daily, which were reviewed by a specialist nurse in another part of the county". The hospital was, in early 2024, looking after 37 patients (with a range of conditions) in virtual beds. The hospital's medical director said: "Each and every one of those patients would ordinarily be in a [hospital] bed, which is a significant percentage of our beds for people who are acutely unwell". In contrast, other doctors suggest that "there's not really evidence at any kind of scale that they're going to relieve the pressures on acute hospitals or are a magic bullet for the much wider system problems".[12]

12. Source of all quotes in this paragraph: www.theguardian.com/society/2024/feb/07/how-virtual-nhs-wards-now-reality

Any health innovation needs to demonstrate improved population health benefits and we need a critical perspective to counter the celebratory accounts. Hendl and Shukla (2024) ask: can digital health democratize healthcare? In their important critique these authors locate such questions in the wider context of global health inequalities, raising "concerns of (data)colonialism, problematizing methodologically white and western design that merely represents and often overlooks and excludes non-western and indigenous populations and their concerns of health and well-being" (493). They argue that "debates on the transformation of healthcare through digital health ought to move beyond democratization toward justice and decolonization, in nonmetaphorical and material terms" (493).

More locally, studies on the use of digital technologies within the US have ignored gender and racial differences, basing their research either exclusively on white people or only male participants (see the comments on AI, above, pp. 15–16). More broadly, we could see the "personalization" of healthcare as redolent of a neoliberal discourse that foregrounds the individual "consumer" who is wholly reliant on a marketplace of apps and mobile devices.

Setting aside these important philosophical questions, what empirical evidence is there that it is inclusive and provided and accessed in an equitable way? Consider first some studies conducted in Sweden. Wilkens *et al.* (2024) compared digital primary care contacts with office-based visits made by adults (a sample of over three-quarters of a million Swedes) in 2018, in order to see if these differed according to income level. About 84 per cent made only office visits, 14 per cent only digital "visits" and a small percentage used both. They found that poorer patients were more likely to make office visits while wealthier and better-educated ones made more use of online services. Rural dwellers were, perhaps surprisingly, under-represented in the digital group (Table 7.2). As the authors put it "There is a contradiction in that rural and elderly patients, who ought to have the most to gain from digital services due to its travel-free nature, were using them less than others" (Wilkens *et al.* 2024: 7–8). Reduced usage among poorer and older patients is no doubt due either to lack of affordable broadband access or lack of

Table 7.2 Comparison of office-based and digital primary care contacts in Sweden

Variable	*Office-based contacts*	*Digital contacts*
Annual gross income (Swedish krona)	267,000	921,000
Patients in sample (%)	83.7	14.2
Women (%)	56.1	65.4
University educated (%)	30.3	52.3
Rural dwelling (%)	23.3	4.8
Unemployed (%)	45.6	14.3

Source: Wilkens *et al.* (2024).

confidence in using it, or both. The conclusion is that, in Sweden at least, the provision of digital services is inequitable.

Telemedicine embraces different media, from telephone calls to video ones – the latter of course mimicking in-person meetings. We might expect the Covid-19 pandemic to have led to increased use of digital healthcare, given restrictions on movement. Here, evidence suggests that people of colour, and older people in the US, made less use of video calls than others. For example, in a study based on haematology appointments in Boston Osei *et al.* (2023) found that while 31 per cent of white patients had video calls only 22 per cent of Black and 19 per cent of Latino patients did so. The authors caution that since "video visits typically offer better clinical interaction than telephone, the observed disparity may exacerbate underlying health inequities if not addressed" (Osei *et al.* 2023: 1270). This finding is mirrored in a study of people experiencing palliative care, where men, Spanish-speakers and uninsured people were significantly less likely to access video calls (Frydman *et al.* 2022).

We noted in Chapter 2 that one dimension of "access" was acceptability: how a service is perceived. People need to be able to trust a clinician with whom they are consulting. To that end it is instructive to note what Yee and colleagues (2022: e480) have to say. "In a discipline like medicine, which is equally humanistic as it is technical, both physical and emotional care are necessary to achieve optimal health outcomes and bolster patient–clinician relationships". They argue that "a more empathetic, patient-centred focus in the current deployment of telemedicine" is required in order to counteract the lack of take-up of telemedicine among currently excluded groups, particularly Black Americans. This argument is developed further by Kepper *et al.* (2024) who suggest the need for behavioural approaches to help understand the take-up of digital healthcare. Yet they stress this requires behavioural change not only by individuals but also providers of care and wider health systems. In particular, healthcare system users need to be involved in design and evaluation. "Equity of digital health tools is improved by undergoing usability testing by diverse, underserved individuals, including those of different generations" (Kepper *et al.* 2024: 6).

But "usability testing" first assumes that there is adequate access to the technology (devices, internet access and so on); if the material infrastructure is missing then digital healthcare is a non-starter. To that end it is instructive to consider the situation in Brazil as described by Nakayama *et al.* (2023) who use data from a survey of almost 280,000 households. There are regional differences in internet usage, with higher prevalence in the South and Southeast than the North and Northeast (Figure 5.2), a divide that mirrors many socio-economic indicators (Gatrell 2023: 30–2). In the North and Northeast regions, the most common reasons for low usage were the lack of internet availability and the cost of internet access. Such regional disparities are clearly a barrier to accessing digital healthcare. In Nigeria, Jennings and colleagues (2015) show that, after controlling for factors such as age and education, in comparison to women who had mobile phones those without made significantly less use of antenatal care and effective contraception. Clearly, if we are to improve maternal healthcare in resource-poor settings it is essential to provide the means to do so digitally (and without relying on male permission; see Scott *et al.* 2021).

In countries of the Global North the issue may be less to do with the availability of digital infrastructure and devices, and more to do with utilization. Zhang *et al.* (2023) explore this in the context of the UK's NHS where there are two universally available digital health interventions: a smartphone application (known as "NHS App") for accessing healthcare services, and a means of contacting primary care (general practices) via a mobile phone. Those living in the most deprived areas of England were significantly less likely to use the App and the primary care "portals" than those in more affluent areas. As the authors wryly note: these "findings are concerning as the NHS aims to make apps the 'front door' to healthcare" (Zhang *et al.* 2023: 2).

In terms of a "patient-centred" perspective it is productive to consider an autoethnographic approach to understanding the "place" of digital health, and Thompson (2021) provides a valuable example, albeit writing (as she acknowledges) as a digitally "comfortable" consumer of healthcare. Thompson has several concerns, not least that it is impossible for the digital user to track how data moves through cyberspace and becomes available to other agencies; if so, technology that should be empowering leaves the client disempowered instead. She acknowledges its value in mental healthcare where "talking therapies" are essential but if technologies (such as Zoom) fail then the "rhythms" of interaction, and the subsequent delivery of care, can be disrupted.

Moving medicines

People and technologies are not the only mobile things. The trade in pharmaceutical products can reinforce inequities in access to potentially life-saving therapies.

In Europe, between 2023 and 2024 imports from the United States decreased by just over 2 per cent while exports increased by 30 per cent. This led to an increase in the trade surplus in Europe from €45 billion in 2023 to €74 billion in 2024. In 2023, the US imported $203 billion in pharmaceutical products, much of these from Europe (notably, Ireland, Germany and Switzerland). The US exported $100 billion in pharmaceutical products in 2023, with major destinations including Germany, Belgium and China. The trade deficit led President Trump to impose tariffs on these products; to avoid these, major firms have pledged billions of dollars of investment in the US.

Statistics on international trade balances tell us nothing about the impacts that such trade have on patient health and safety. Not all products that are shipped across the globe are safe (Box 7.3).

BOX 7.3 SHIPPING POOR-QUALITY DRUGS

The treatment of acute lymphoblastic leukaemia (ALL) in children involves using a drug called asparaginase. However, in low- and middle-income countries access to this medicine is limited and substandard preparations of asparaginase – distributed from China and India – have been marketed in many African countries (especially Uganda, Ghana and Malawi). The impact of such poor-quality drugs has been profound, the problem emerging first in Brazil in 2017 when the brand Leuginase – coming from a pharmaceutical company in Beijing – was found to be contaminated. In addition, seven Indian companies who were warned about their defective preparations of asparaginase continued to market the product internationally. Further investigation suggests that "lax regulation and oversight has allowed these products to proliferate, and little has been done to increase access to high-quality drugs for the world's poorest".[13]

Higher prices for different drugs to treat ALL mean that they are unaffordable in many low- and middle-income countries. For example, one brand, Oncaspar, cost $1,700 in 2015 but when pharmaceutical companies merged its price increased to $18,000.

The Bureau of Investigative Journalism reports that:

> Roughly 10% of medicines sold in low and middle-income countries are thought to be fake or substandard, with tragic consequences. In October, the deaths of nearly 70 children in Gambia were linked to an Indian-made cough syrup. Last month, 18 children died in Uzbekistan after taking another Indian-made cough syrup. Fixing the systemic issues that have allowed poor-quality asparaginase to spread could help patients far beyond child cancer wards.
>
> *(ibid.)*

For further details, see Barr *et al.* (2023).

Miller and colleagues (2021) have explored the rise in "e-pharmacy" – using the internet to sell medicines – and consider the impact this has for low- and middle-income countries. Its fast-growing expansion is, they assert, largely uncontrolled, with worrying issues including the marketing of medicines that ought only to be prescribed by a health professional, and the lack of information accompanying the sale. Set against these concerns are better access to drugs for those living in areas that are poorly served by pharmacy

13. www.thebureauinvestigates.com/stories/2023-01-25/the-drug-was-meant-to-save-childrens-lives-instead-theyre-dying/

outlets. Miller *et al.* (2021: 4) highlight some obvious concerns, such as the over-use of antibiotics (leading to antimicrobial resistance) and opioids, as well as the "challenge of using national regulatory frameworks to control a market that operates with ease across geographical boundaries". Stopping counterfeit drugs remains a challenge but improved labelling and the use of technologies such as holograms and QR codes helps authenticate drug packaging.

Concluding remarks

Many discussions of access to healthcare focus – as we have seen in previous chapters – on the utilization of such care at fixed sites: clinics and hospitals. Accessing these necessarily involves movement: getting from the home to a healthcare facility, for example. In a sense, all healthcare involves mobility, whether of patient, healthcare professional or the materials needed for care. "Mobilities" has been something of a leitmotif running through the book, but within this the key theme has been one of equity. In examining what, and who, moves we have seen that some people are constrained in their access to healthcare, while others are simply denied it. For some population groups (travellers, for example) their very nomadic existence makes access challenging. For others, notably refugees, the sedentarist nature of healthcare provision at fixed sites places barriers on access, while international borders render access deeply problematic.

This chapter has also examined alternative forms of access, including the provision and use of mobile facilities, and the use of telehealthcare. Even here there are issues of equity of provision and use. Ironically, those subgroups that might benefit most from care – particularly those in rural communities far removed from clinics and hospitals – seem often to lack the material infrastructure (such as fast broadband) that would enable virtual access. It remains to be seen how far digital healthcare diffuses across the globe and whether it leads to more equitable healthcare.

We have also examined health or medical "tourism" and the equity dimensions to this. While the financial costs of seeking care abroad may be significantly less than at home, such travel may be impossible for some. In addition, we noted how the host population cannot hope in many circumstances to access the surgery or other treatment that they too might require but which is well beyond their means.

Put simply, there are significant mobility *constraints* on accessing healthcare, whether because of travel time or cost or availability of infrastructure. While innovative forms of service delivery can help ensure access for some remote or disadvantaged populations this too is patterned socially, with some missing out on care that may be desperately needed.

Further reading

On the subject of mobilities there is now an extensive literature, as well as at least two academic journals devoted to it; these are *Mobilities*[14] and *Applied Mobilities.*[15]

A good starting point is the collection of essays edited by Adey *et al.* (2017), but with respect to healthcare see the chapters in Follis *et al.* (2025).

Connell & Walton-Roberts (2016) have an excellent review of research on the mobilities of skilled health workers.

On medical tourism see Connell (2011) for a critical perspective, with particular reference to Thailand, but also Malaysia and India. Smith (2012) is an excellent read but see also her book on medical tourism to India (Smith 2022). Chapter 13 in Brown *et al.* (2018) is also very useful.

On technology-enabled care in the home, see Reid (2021).

14. www.tandfonline.com/journals/rmob20
15. www.tandfonline.com/journals/rapm20

8

WHO CARES IN THE COMMUNITY?

> The division of responsibility between the state's own "'market" of care, the private sector and the family can vary significantly from country to country on account of different ideological, cultural and political debates.
>
> Power (2018: 95)

To care (the verb) means "feeling concern or taking an interest" (as in "I care about what government gets elected"). Throughout this book we have invariably looked at care as a noun – the work involved in attending to someone in need of clinical assessment and then providing necessary treatment. It is time to examine the verb rather than the noun. There is a vast literature on this topic, including much written by geographers, but in keeping with the book's general theme I focus where possible on the inequalities or inequities in provision and utilization.

What follows examines, first, care given in the home, next residential care (assisted living) and care during the Covid-19 pandemic, before turning to the role of volunteering. Given the ageing population in most countries in the Global North, such caregiving is often for older adults and this is the main focus, acknowledging that other care is given to younger people with disabilities and to children. But we should note that for some writers, especially those concerned with disability, the words "support" and "personal assistance" are preferred to "care", since they are less suggestive of dependency (Power 2018: 108).

While this chapter refers to care "*in* the community" such care is, rather, provided "*by* the community" (Power 2018: 99), confirming that much of the provision is undertaken by the informal and voluntary sectors, rather than the state. To that end, as well as discussing the informal care provided by family members, we discuss – with a critical eye – the role of the voluntary sector in providing care, in both the Global North and Global South.

Care in the home

Large-scale restructuring of healthcare systems in many countries in the Global North has taken some care out of the hospital setting and into the home (see Box 8.1). Hospital managers are invariably keen to discharge patients into the "community"; what that means is shifting care into residential or nursing homes or to the private space of the home where usually it is women who undertake the (unpaid) labour of care. It also absolves the state from having to adequately fund services, in keeping with austerity programmes set up in the neoliberal era (see Brown *et al.* 2010: 567–86).

BOX 8.1 TRANSITIONING FROM HOSPITAL TO HOME OR RESIDENTIAL CARE

The previous chapter discussed "mobilities" in relation to healthcare. One important such example concerns the challenges of moving ("discharging") patients out of hospital either back home or to a nursing or residential home. The challenges arise if the patient no longer requires clinical care in the hospital and is well enough to be discharged, yet there is nowhere for them to go. Commonly, and regrettably, this is referred to as "bed blocking" in the UK, but this suggests the fault lies with the patient rather than the care system. It is preferable to speak of "delayed transfer of care". Hinde *et al.* (2021) suggested that, in England in 2014–15 about 2.7 billion bed-days were occupied by older people who no longer required acute hospital care. This reflects the lack of coordination between the health service and social care services. There are knock-on effects on accident and emergency services in hospitals, which become overcrowded if there are no in-patient beds available for those admitted to A&E and in need of such. There is a geography to this. Gaughan *et al.* (2015) found that in England while an increase in care home beds in local authorities reduced delayed discharges, there were "spillover effects". A greater availability of care home beds in nearby areas were associated with fewer delayed discharges.

It is helpful to think of this issue in terms of "assemblage", with a range of actors (hospital managers, care homes, clinicians, carers, patients and so on) coming together to try to manage discharge. Similarly, others have drawn on Bourdieu's concept of the "field", "which embraces the various structures, institutions, authorities and activities people act within … the field is comprised of the transitional care services for older people from hospital to home via intermediate care" (Kvæl & Gautun 2023). As noted in Chapter 2 there are various strands of "capital" (economic, social, cultural) on which patients might (or might not) be able to draw to affect discharge; but these are subject to health and social care organizational constraints. In their study of transitions from hospital to home in Norway Kvæl and Gautun (2023) find that "navigating the healthcare maze depends on where you live, your levels of education and health literacy and your ability to mobilize social networks". Different amounts and forms of capital shape access to care services.

Such a change in provision has consequences for carers' (particularly women's) own health and well-being, as well as implications for any paid employment they have. A good example of this comes from a study undertaken by Brassolotto and Daly (2016). These authors adopt the framework of feminist political economy to explore the care given in the home to people on dialysis (for renal disease). Such demanding work has implications for those doing the caring, including sacrificing their own hobbies and neglecting their own health. The author's specific focus is rural British Columbia, where centralization of services has placed more of the care burden on the domestic environment and women in particular. While some training on home dialysis is available, this hardly compensates for the lengthy training that health professionals receive. Further, those on very low incomes could not afford respite care, paid companions or assistance from the private sector. The authors' feminist political economy lens illustrates that "a consequence of shifting treatment from the clinic to the home is the substantial amount of invisible work, costs, and responsibility transferred from institutions to patients and their families" (Brassolotto & Daly 2016: 528). In similar research in Canada Holland (2022) refers to the "invisible" work undertaken by carers; such work "is not limited to specific tasks but includes the mental and emotional, invisible labour required in navigating the home as a health care environment and government programs designed, ostensibly, to ease their burden" (Holland 2022: 1). Moreover, the burdens fall more heavily on those with less economic capital. "Families with lower household incomes experienced barriers to negotiating with the home space for the purpose of health work because they lacked resources to make necessary repairs and 'push back' on the encroaching institutionalized look and feel of the home" (Holland 2022: 6).

Research by Wiles (2003) reveals how the poor mobility of the person being cared for constrains the mobility of the caregiver themselves. She documents how caring is both physically and emotionally draining. Mobility is place-dependent; while some people needing support can negotiate home space quite confidently it is a different matter out of the house. The nature of the home space depends on income; wealthier people can afford to modify the domestic space or buy mobility aids that others might find too costly. Social capital (networks of others who can provide domestic help and support) as well as economic and mobility capital (above, pp. 26–8) benefits both caregiver and recipient. Access to healthcare outside the home is also challenging. "Caregivers described having to wait lengthy times at health appointments. Many of the people receiving care had several doctor, specialist, and other visits in a week, and caregivers spent a great deal of time co-ordinating these appointments and then waiting for them" (Wiles 2003: 1321).

These issues are not restricted to the Global North. Studies have revealed that family caregivers report considerable stresses as a result of the need to provide social, economic and emotional support, not least to those living with chronic infections. For example, in their study of those giving care to family members living with AIDS in Uganda Kipp *et al.* (2007: 1) write: "As the requirements for family care giving are often overwhelming for women under the conditions as they exist in Uganda and in other developing countries, it constitutes a gender issue of great importance that has not been appreciated fully in the international literature". Kohli *et al.* (2012) document similar findings in India. Home care for people living with HIV was much preferred (both by them and their caregivers) to hospital-based care, where costs (including transport) and risks of stigmatization were a concern. Again, women bore the brunt of care: "Women provided unconditional support to their HIV positive spouses even if it meant having a sexual relationship" (Kohli *et al.* 2012: 5). Women were caregivers, regardless of their own health status.

Some researchers have explored the usefulness of the concept of therapeutic landscapes (above, pp. 9–10) for those needing care in the home. For example, English and her colleagues (2008) signalled the importance of the home environment in providing care for survivors of, or recently diagnosed with, breast cancer. Specific centres in Toronto explored in that research provide art and music therapy, as well as alternative therapies offering hope and healing. Research too on natural landscapes (e.g. Milligan & Bingley 2007) suggests that care – in its broadest sense – can take place outside the clinical setting as well as in such settings themselves (see, e.g., Hjort *et al.* 2023). Further, while it is now widely accepted that green spaces (parks, woodland and so on) confer health benefits, geographic access to these is inequitable (see, e.g., Miller *et al.* 2022). However, while the home may be a "therapeutic landscape" for the patient, it is less so for the caregiver, for whom the home can be a site of stress and struggle, reflecting the labour (physical and emotional) involved. In addition, the caregiver may be forgoing employment (and therefore income) for a period, making the work health-detracting and certainly not therapeutic.

These "struggles" beg the question as to what role can be played by telehealthcare (above, pp. 157–61), which embraces a range of digital telecommunication devices and assistive technologies, including sensors that can detect movement (and potential falls) and communicate remotely with external agencies (Milligan *et al.* 2011). These may sit alongside simpler technologies such as mobile phones and personal computers but these are hardly "simple" for users who are visually and/or cognitively impaired, or constrained by other chronic physical conditions. When they are usable, they can provide a degree of independence and maintain – often at considerable distances – social connectedness, albeit without direct human contact and companionship. As Hwang *et al.* (2024) put it (with their emphasis on the use of AI) we can envisage technology "to be more than a tool, but rather a relational and felt experience, through which actors shape, and are shaped, by their interactions". How these experiences might change, and for whom, as quite sophisticated "care robots" become more widely used is a moot point.

A critical analysis needs to ask how these technologies re-model the home environment and if they perpetuate inequalities. Milligan *et al.* (2011) have argued that their introduction serves to blur the boundaries between the home and institutional space. The impetus given to these technologies by governments informed by a neoliberal agenda with its focus on austerity is intended to reduce the burden on over-stretched healthcare providers (as well as the shortage of social care places). Some critics argue that the technologies cannot substitute for human contact. As one respondent (Milligan *et al.* 2011: 350) puts it:

> *Technology can never replace human contact and carers. Carers come to [my wife] and I think apart from the practical things that they do for her, I hear laughter going on all the time in the social interaction. And the laughter – that's so important and cannot be replaced by technology.*

As this suggests, such technologies are never used in isolation; relationships between users, carers and clinicians are crucial if they are to be successful.

Such relationships are key to the "Hospital at Home" model. This is "an acute clinical service that takes staff, equipment, technologies, medication and skills usually provided in hospitals and delivers that hospital care to *selected people* in their homes or in nursing homes" (my italics)[1] (see Figure 8.1). The key here is "selected people" – does this refer to clinical need or some personal attributes such as wealth or class?

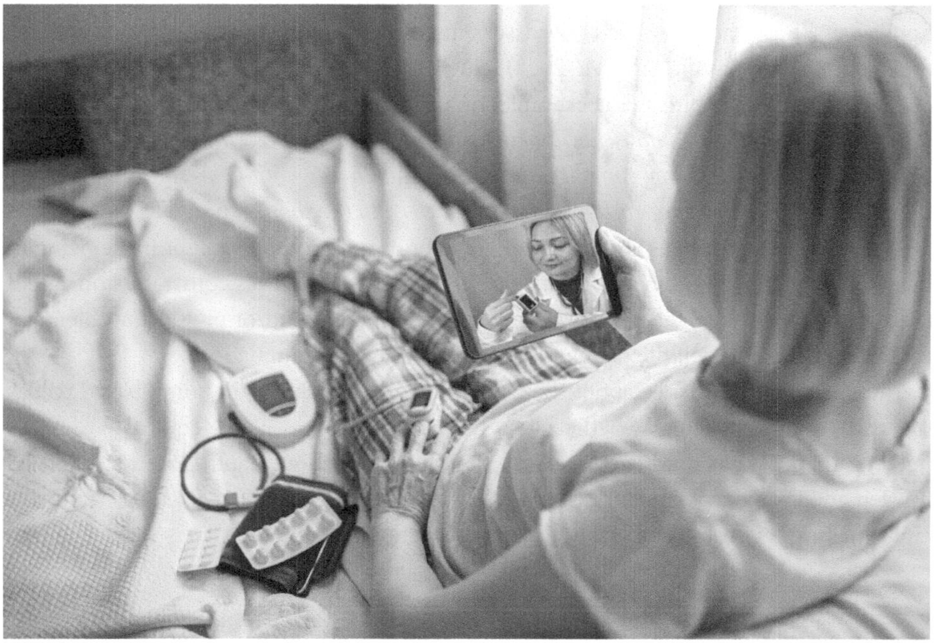

Figure 8.1 Telehealthcare: "Hospital at Home"
Source: iStock ID:1295613094.

1. www.hospitalathome.org.uk

One advantage of a formal "hospital at home" (HaH) arrangement over a less formalized presence of digital and other technologies in the home is that, as Siu *et al.* (2022: 3) put it, a visiting clinician can actually "directly observe and provide care to patients in their homes, where they can address social determinants of health (e.g., food insecurity, medical equipment needs, management of chronic diseases in real-world situations)". Because of this the authors suggest that HaH has at least as many benefits for socio-economically disadvantaged patients as for better-off ones. Yet in the US there is an unequal geography, with most services provided in urban areas where HaH staff can reach the home relatively easily, compared with rural areas where they have further to travel. Further, not all states provide funding for HaH services – California is one that does not.

In Chapter 4 we considered access to palliative care, but the focus was very much on access to hospices. Yet some palliative care is delivered to patients at home; many people nearing the end of life have a strong preference to die at home rather than in a hospital. What is known about the inequalities here?

Quinn *et al.* (2023: 2) note that "inequities in access and experience of palliative care appear to operate along the same social divisions as other forms of privilege, including ethnicity, gender, age, disability status and access to financial resources and the intersections between these". In their study of the behaviour of palliative care nurses' home visits the authors revealed how assessments were made of material circumstances of patients, noting (as did Sui *et al.* 2022) "clues" that would signal if people were experiencing financial difficulties. For example, one Scottish nurse has this to say about her patient: "*Unkempt, you know, not looking after themselves, very frail, food that's been in the fridge for a long, long time, it's all out of date. There's nothing fresh because either they haven't got to the shop, or they can't afford to go to the shop*" (quoted in Quinn *et al.* 2023: 5). For poor people, the rising costs of energy and food bills might make being in hospital a preferable option. But the layout of the home too places constraints on care if there is limited space to accommodate medical equipment and/or physical problems of accessing the property if the patient lives in high-rise accommodation.

There is limited evidence about the use of digital technologies in home-based palliative care and in particular whether such technologies are available equitably to those needing them. What does seem clear is that concerns about digital "literacy" and its uneven adoption may be misplaced. Older adults engaged in palliative care are, in principle, increasingly comfortable with the use of technological tools.

Residential care homes

Those requiring care outside the hospital or home may find themselves in residential care homes or settings offering significant nursing care. Between these we can speak of "assisted living", where there might be some supportive services shared between residents living in their own rooms or apartments. In principle this can lead to new social relationships and a sense of community based on shared interests and activities (such as gardening). As Cutchin (2007) notes, the concept of therapeutic landscapes is relevant here too, although it should not be applied uncritically. As we saw with how hospitals can present themselves (above, pp. 9–10) some care homes project images, often unrealistic, about what it is like to live there. Such images "present commodities of the landscape that are of particular interest to persons of higher socioeconomic class with particular cultural backgrounds and tastes" (Cutchin 2007: 189). Further, "transitioning" from one's own home to an entirely new setting means that the social connections may be a struggle to realize.

While the state – at least in the Global North – may provide some financial support for residential care, the cost of this often falls on the individuals and families involved. This means that some such care is "top of the range" while other settings may lack the ambience and quality of the provision that is available to the better-off. In some places the range of activities on offer and the quality of care provided may be rather modest, even perfunctory. At the extreme, we often hear stories of older adults, and those with intellectual disabilities, being physically and emotionally abused. Much abuse is likely to go unreported. Some of it reflects lack of staff, poor training and supervision, but also residents' behaviour, which can be directed at other residents; see Hirt and colleagues (2022) for a recent overview. In July 2024 the BBC reported on the state of care homes in England, noting that the Care Quality Commission (CQC, the body regulating care homes) found that one in five such homes were rated as "requiring improvement" or (worse) "inadequate".[2]

We noted in earlier chapters the ways in which healthcare in the Global North is being privatized. The same is happening in social care, with provision shifting from the state to the private (often, for-profit) sector. In England almost 90 per cent of adult social care provision is run by the private, for-profit sector (Bach-Mortensen *et al.* 2024). These authors note that "for-profit care homes deliver worse quality than public and third sector (non-profit) care homes ... the pursuit of profit influences the behaviour of providers in ways that negatively impact the quality of care" (Bach-Mortensen *et al.* 2024: 2; see also Bach-Mortensen *et al.* 2025). In the US, there is evidence that the quality of care services is worse in areas of deprivation, a finding confirmed in England where for-profit care home inspection ratings (by the CQC) are worst in the most deprived areas (Bach-Mortensen *et al.* 2024).

In the US, long-term services and support (LTSS) refers to personal care that is delivered in the community or at home. It "is highly variable across local geographies; services are typically arranged by individuals and families and subject to state and local

2. www.bbc.co.uk/news/articles/c4ngegrlwvgo

health policies and resources within a fractured United States welfare and health care system" (Fabius *et al.* 2023: 1078). As a result, there is variability in terms of access and quality. Fabius and colleagues found that adverse consequences resulting from unmet needs were more common for older adults living in areas of poverty or poor social cohesion. In earlier research Mor *et al.* (2004) found that nursing homes with residents who were highly dependent on Medicaid for funding were more likely to have fewer, less qualified, registered nurses per resident, while residents received poorer care. Specifically, the incidence of pressure ulcers and use of physical restraints were more common in "lower tier" homes (those with high percentages of Medicaid residents).

Elsewhere, research has confirmed both the difficulties in recruiting care home staff to poorly paid positions and the increasing reliance on migrant workers, whose working conditions are challenging. Simmons *et al.* (2022) have explored this issue, using surveys of about 1,800 care staff (both migrant and non-migrant) to compare working conditions in Austria and Sweden. Migrant workers reported more stress, and both physical and mental exhaustion, in Sweden than in Austria, with non-European migrants complaining of racist treatment. Further, while one-fifth of migrant workers in Austria said they wanted to leave their work, twice as many in Sweden wanted to quit their job. This is partly explained by the differences in provision. In Sweden, the private sector consists of mainly large, for-profit companies, while in Austria the private sector comprises mostly non-profit organizations.

Care for those living with disability

One billion people around the world live with disabilities, a leading report suggesting that they are being "left behind" in studies of global health.[3] People with disabilities include those with long-term physical, mental, intellectual, developmental or sensory impairments (such as hearing and vision loss). They are often on low incomes and lacking the employment opportunities afforded to non-disabled people. These inequalities are compounded by poor access to good quality healthcare, with many of the same issues (such as high transport costs, long waiting times for medical appointments and too short consultation times) that affect non-disabled people also affecting disabled access. Yet the healthcare needs may be more significant, including the costs of specialized equipment or assistive technologies. Similarly, disabled people (especially those with intellectual and developmental disabilities in non-metropolitan areas) have poorer access to healthcare services and preventive healthcare utilization (Gréaux *et al.* 2023).

3. www.lshtm.ac.uk/media/38726

Taking cancer screening as an example, research suggests that people with disabilities have lower rates of cancer screening. Keegan *et al.* (2023) report that women with a disability have a 22 per cent lower likelihood of having regular breast screening compared with non-disabled women. For women with mobility issues the lack of accessible screening equipment (that is, at a suitable height) is a major barrier since mammography is invariably performed in a standing position. But there are other structural factors at work. Uninsured disabled people have poorer access to care than do people with disabilities who have insurance. White women with intellectual disabilities are significantly more likely to have mammograms, compared with Black women with the same disabilities. Geography matters too: women with a disability who live in rural settings are less likely to be screened, either for breast or cervical cancer. In a US study between 2002 and 2008 Horner-Johnson *et al.* (2015) showed that while 84.4 per cent of rural-living women without a disability had received cervical cancer screening, only 74.4 per cent of women with a disability had. Comparable figures for mammography were 70.2 and 67.3 respectively. The authors suggest that, in rural areas, "doctors' offices may be in older, less accessible buildings and women have fewer options when attempting to locate an accessible clinic" (Horner-Johnson *et al.* 2015: 251).

The review by Greaux and colleagues (2023) reveals that healthcare workers are sometimes inexperienced in dealing with people with disabilities, and some are guilty of discriminatory attitudes and unacceptable behaviours. From time to time there are reports of bullying (including online "trolling"[4]) and violent behaviour.[5]

The *Missing Billion* report (Kuper & Heydt 2019) asserts that poor access to healthcare services is a violation of the rights of people with disabilities; further, in a global context such poor access means that the key components of universal healthcare coverage (pp. 85–7 above) – coverage of services, appropriate services and affordability – will not be achievable. Globally, "half of people with disabilities cannot afford healthcare, and they are 50 per cent more likely to experience catastrophic health expenditure" (Kuper & Heydt 2019: 9). Further, in parts of Africa (Kenya and Malawi, for example) services to improve hearing impairment are not publicly funded but rely on charitable donations.

Generalizations are fraught with danger, and to lump together "disabled people" as a homogeneous category is unacceptable. Hearing stories about poor access is fruitful and Anon (2024) offers a compelling example of a woman with intellectual disabilities (Box 8.2).

4. www.scope.org.uk/media/press-releases/scope-reveals-shocking-levels-of-online-trolling-experienced-by-disabled-people
5. www.learningdisabilitytoday.co.uk/news/cqc-puts-kent-care-home-into-special-measures-following-abuse-and-safeguarding-failures/

BOX 8.2 EQUITY OF ACCESS TO HEALTHCARE FOR PATIENTS WITH INTELLECTUAL DISABILITIES

Dorothy [a pseudonym] has a severe intellectual disability (Anon 2024). She lives, with others who have such disabilities, in a care home where she and others are supported by staff. The author tells us that it is deeply problematic for her to access the healthcare she needs, whether this be dental care, checking her blood pressure or other preventive care. She is nervous around doctors and nurses, and resists any physical investigations. She has difficulties voicing her needs and her wishes. As with others living with intellectual disabilities there were particular problems when she was due to receive her first Covid-19 vaccine. She was unable to give informed consent and could not attend the clinic; she required sedation in order to relax and manage the vaccination. This leads the author to ask: "What else can be done while she is sedated? Blood tests for hormonal changes? Blood pressure checks? Optometry? Audiology? Would it be possible to set up a regular multidisciplinary one-stop-shop?"

Since Dorothy and others in a similar situation are unable to express their needs there are significant and complex barriers to healthcare access.

Setting this in a wider context, Lincoln *et al.* (2023) contrast the vaccinations given in different world regions. In early 2022, in high income countries about 94 per cent of people with intellectual disabilities had been vaccinated, compared with 61 per cent in lower-middle income countries and just 38 per cent in low-income countries. Poor access to vaccination clinics was an issue, echoing the issues for non-disabled populations.

Care during the Covid-19 pandemic

There are plenty of stories about accessing care during the Covid-19 pandemic. For many people the absence of human contact was deeply distressing, particularly for those living in care homes where their family members were unable to visit. There is a wealth of evidence concerning mortality in care homes and how those people living in care homes were impacted significantly by the pandemic, in terms of social and physical isolation. Noting the strictures of Connell and Walton-Roberts (2016; see above, pp. 146–7) concerning the lack of geographic attention given to the healthcare workforce we consider this issue briefly in relation to inequality.

More than 1.6 million people work in adult social care across Britain, and in general this is a lower-paid workforce. In 2019–20, almost three-quarters of those working in adult social care in the independent sector in England were paid less than the "living wage" (£9.30 per hour in 2020, £10.55 in London). Women made up over 80 per cent

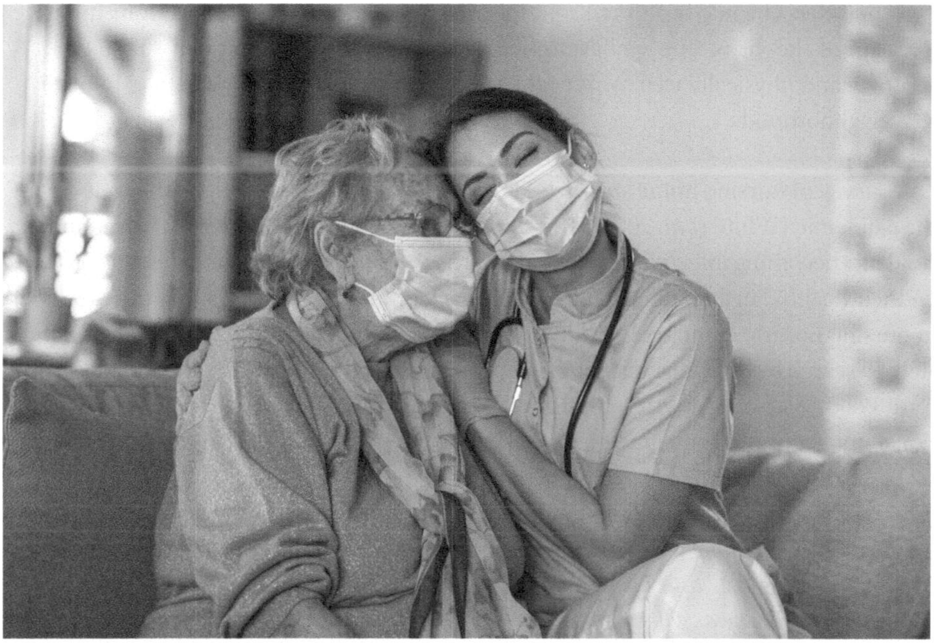

Figure 8.2 Home care visit to an older adult during the Covid-19 pandemic
Source: iStock ID:1295992218.

of that workforce (Figure 8.2). Ethnic minority workers (notably Black people) reported racism or discrimination at work and were invariably unsupported by line managers. This was particularly acute during the pandemic. Some ethnic minority social care workers highlighted shortages of suitable personal protective equipment (PPE) as the Covid-19 pandemic took hold.[6]

As is well known, social interaction during the pandemic had to be at-a-distance, with people separated by doors and windows, or it had to be provided remotely in order to ensure some form of human contact. In Arkansas, United States, medical students from the university in Little Rock set up a "Geriatric Buddy" scheme, where volunteers met older care home residents on Zoom or FaceTime, to simply chat or play games or help solve puzzles online. Geriatrician Priya Mendiratta, MD who led the programme explained the reasons for it:

> Our experience in the past has taught us that social isolation in the elderly puts them at risk for further cognitive decline, worsening of depression and anxiety

6. www.equalityhumanrights.com/our-work/inquiries-and-investigations/experiences-health-and-social-care-treatment-lower-paid

> and other chronic health risks. ... Isolating the elderly might reduce transmission of the virus, but we have to look into strategies to help them stay mentally and physically well. ... We all need to reach out to older neighbors in our neighborhoods.[7]

A survey of nursing home staff in 32 US states explored the emotions they felt during the pandemic (White *et al.* 2021). They expressed anxiety about both themselves and the residents becoming infected, as well as concerns about the impact of increased workloads on their health. Further, they bemoaned the lack of media coverage about the situations in nursing homes, compared with the "heroic" public recognition accorded to hospital staff. Research by the University of Exeter, and published by the International Long Term Care Policy Network in 2022 confirmed these findings.[8] The study explored the emotional impact of the pandemic on care home workers in the UK. Workers used military metaphors to describe their experiences. One said:

> *I recall going home once and my husband said to me, "You're going to die if you don't have a rest," and I said to him, "If I die I die," because I could not leave the residents. That was when people needed me most ... It's like somebody in the army. When a war breaks out you don't say, "I'm going to rest." You have to give your life. Life on the frontline, isn't it?*

Another reported: "*All of our head office team, who were our support service, no longer could come into the home because they were on lockdown ... the drawbridge was pulled up from every angle*". Set against these emotions was the resilience shown by employees and a strong sense of teamwork.

Evidence from England and Wales during the pandemic suggested that it had a major impact on people working in the social care sector; the standardized mortality rate in that sector was twice that of the general population.[9] Several factors may have been at play. Workers in the social care sector are on low pay and insecure contracts. Shortages of PPE were widely reported. Close physical proximity among staff and patients made the circulation of the virus much more likely.

7. www.aha.org/other-resources/2020-11-11-geriatric-buddy-program-eases-social-isolation-during-COVID-19
8. https://ltcCOVID.org/wp-content/uploads/2020/12/COVID-impact-on-care-staff-wellbeing-Full-report.pdf
9. www.health.org.uk/features-and-opinion/features/what-has-been-the-impact-of-COVID-19-on-care-homes-and-the-social

Volunteering care

In principle, there is a role for people in the community – aside from family members discussed above – to volunteer their time either to deliver health and social care or to point people in need to the right sources of such care. In the UK there are various local schemes in operation, as noted by Helpforce, an umbrella group that "works with partners across health, care and the community, to develop and evaluate services that optimize the difference volunteers can make".[10] Many local schemes are linked with NHS hospitals, as in London where there is "a fantastic opportunity for volunteers to raise people's awareness of the offers that the Trust provides to local communities, helping them to access care services more easily". Such "offers" include "direct engagement with residents in the community, as they visit them at local libraries or places of worship".[11] Of course, what such volunteering does is to substitute for what the state might otherwise provide. Austerity programmes (above, pp. 53–5) and associated cutbacks in state welfare provision have left gaps in care that volunteers can fill.

On a much broader scale we can consider the role played by International Voluntary Health Networks (IVHNs) that connect relatively rich and poor countries. Such networks are explored critically by Reid *et al.* (2018). Drawing on concepts of capital (see Chapter 2) borrowed from Bourdieu, these authors suggest that international voluntary healthcare workers are engaged in processes of capital exchange whereby they accrue cultural capital through working overseas while those they care for may accrue health capital. Yet the relationship between the volunteer and the person in need is profoundly unequal: one can return to a place of comfort and safety while the other remains poorly located, both geographically and economically.

In similar vein, Herrick and Brooks (2019) examine the roles played by international volunteers during the Ebola epidemic in Sierra Leone, West Africa between 2013 and 2016. The volunteers they consider were British medical students although the authors note that the majority of those volunteering were Sierra Leoneans. One interviewee stated that "*reading in the news about the shortage of healthcare workers and how more manpower was needed on the ground in terms of providing healthcare I figured, well you know if I can be of any service, I would be more than willing to go*" (in Herrick & Brooks 2019: 7). This was a common refrain: students felt they were in a position to offer care and were therefore prepared to do so. As found by Reid and colleagues (2018) there was an accrual of cultural capital, volunteers making firm friends and developing strong contact networks for the future, as well as experiencing an African country, often for the first time.

10. https://helpforce.community/our-services
11. https://helpforce.community/connecting/news-stories/how-volunteers-play-a-vital-part-in-closing-the-gap-on-health-inequality

Other authors suggest that, in delivering care, volunteer doctors have at times done more harm than good. Bauer (2017) documents some such harms. Aside from arrogant behaviours and condescension to those in need of help, there is often inappropriate treatment and little follow-up of patients. Some volunteers may unwittingly create local unemployment because they are providing free services, thereby replacing, albeit temporarily, local clinicians. At worst, this is "self-serving neo-colonialism"; there is a "dark side to international volunteering" (Bauer 2017: 2). Short-term placements of medical students taking electives cannot hope to do anything to address underlying structural inequalities manifest in healthcare systems. Clearly, there are ethical concerns that need to be addressed about these forms of care.

Concluding remarks

As noted earlier (pp. 26–8), the French sociologist Pierre Bourdieu speaks of various social fields or spaces within which social activity takes place. In a range of works (Thomson 2008) he discusses the fields of education, science, television and housing. As noted in this chapter, following Kvæl and Gautun (2023: 6), we can think of "community care" as a field of activity that "embraces the various structures, institutions, authorities and activities people act within". The unequal provision of care in the community is dictated by structural factors such as the nature and level of support provided by the state. However, the impacts of such factors are felt very much at the individual and family level and the burden of care falls invariably, and unequally, on women, whether in countries in the Global North or in the Global South.

This suggests that a structurationist perspective is singularly helpful. While people may be able to exercise choice (agency) in accessing care for older relatives, or disabled family members, they are constrained by organizational structures, whether these be set at national level or more locally. Crucially, people need access to various forms of capital within the community care "field" in order to make decisions about support. To find, and pay for, a good care home for ageing relatives in the Global North requires a significant amount of economic capital, as does the purchase of assistive technologies for a disabled child or partner. Community care requires access to social and cultural capital: whether there are "levers" that can be pulled through different levels of education, health knowledge and ability to draw on family and social networks. Within the home one needs financial capital to purchase the material goods and technologies that enable care to take place in that setting. Stocks of social capital are also needed if one is to remain "connected" to others who can provide emotional and practical support.

It is clear from this chapter that there is inequality in care provision within and outside the home, income and gender intersecting to create such. When we pose the question, "Who cares in the community?" the evidence rather suggests that inequalities in access to such residential care are as much a feature of *social* care as they are of access to *health* care – the main focus of this book.

Further reading

For a good discussion of the geography of care, albeit with a focus on the UK and US, see Power (2018).

The report by Kuper and Heydt (2019) on healthcare access for people with disabilities is an excellent source; it includes useful vignettes about particular individuals and their difficulties in accessing healthcare.

On the effects of Covid-19 (and other crises) on women healthcare workers' health and well-being, see the review by Morgan *et al.* (2022).

9

CONCLUSION

When I started to write this book President Trump had yet to begin a second term in the White House, Russia had yet to invade Ukraine and Gaza had yet to become a site of utter devastation. The healthcare impacts of the Trump presidency have still to be fully manifested, although I have tried in Chapter 3 to offer an interim statement. The healthcare impacts of the humanitarian crisis in Gaza have figured in earlier chapters, but the full human cost of the tragedy will be felt for many years. The outcome of Russia's invasion also remains very uncertain, and research has yet to reveal anything about its impact on the geography of healthcare (although see Węgrzynowska *et al.* 2024 for its impact on maternity services).

Since beginning writing, other issues have emerged, or intensified. Among these I would highlight the growth of artificial intelligence (AI) and the debates around gender identity. Whether the former has consequences for understanding the geography of healthcare access remains to be seen. As for the latter, I have touched on this in Chapter 2, noting the stress involved in accessing helpful and sensitive care if seeking to transition.

These preliminary remarks suggest that writing a set of "conclusions" is fraught with danger. Nonetheless, I attempt to reflect on some of the themes that the book has addressed. These are as follows.

Approaches to understanding access to healthcare

In Chapter 2 I outlined and illustrated various theoretical approaches to understanding the geography of access to healthcare. The approach that one takes depends, of course, on the question being asked or the problem being addressed. If one wishes to estimate the extent to which healthcare facilities are spatially accessible, and to whom, then we need quantitative methods and accurate, detailed spatial data to help us. This kind of work is labelled "positivist", although that is a simplistic label to attach to it (Cresswell 2024: 80–81). In order to understand the barriers that people face in seeking to access healthcare we need to draw on qualitative methods, and a "social interactionist" approach offers more insight, with interviews and focus groups the means to unpack the human agency involved in healthcare decision-making. We must not lose sight of the fact that healthcare is delivered to individual people, whose lives may be rich or impoverished, solitary or embedded in family and social networks, benefiting from interventions of one sort or another, or nearing the end of life. Circumstances and emotions matter.

If we are interested in the "bigger picture" – the provision of healthcare within a wider national and international context – then a political economy or "structuralist" account is required. That requires an analysis of the roles played by international organizations and national governments, and the financial imperatives they impose. Such roles change as new leaders emerge. The consequences of these decisions are felt acutely by individuals and communities, whether in countries of the Global North or South. The healthcare-seeking behaviours of individual actors are therefore shaped by both these "macro-level" decisions and their own knowledge and attitudes. This leads some writers on healthcare to adopt a "structurationist" approach, which argues that decision-making by individuals is set within that wider structural context. We saw how this approach was in essence that adopted by the French sociologist Pierre Bourdieu. In that regard, healthcare is a social "field" involving a range of actors and/or organizations, each of which has different forms and amounts of "capital" that is accumulated and exchanged. Such capital includes economic (financial assets), cultural (knowledge and preferences) and social (family and community ties and networks). To this list we can add "health capital" (whether one enjoys good or less good health), as this very much dictates whether we need to access healthcare, and what form that should take. My own view is that a structurationist perspective is particularly helpful in understanding the social geography of healthcare.

The last perspective mentioned in Chapter 2 was a "poststructuralist" one. Although this umbrella term comprises a range of perspectives, at heart it is "happy to stay at the surface of life rather than digging for further 'truth'" (Cresswell 2024: 209). Further, it stresses the relationality of different elements. We saw that an important concept is "assemblage", a network of things that coalesce. In a healthcare context this includes people (patients, clinicians), technologies and devices (equipment, pharmaceuticals), buildings (clinics, hospitals), and the various means of transport that enable, or constrain, access to healthcare. Access to all elements in such networks is clearly unequal, as we have seen throughout the book.

The meanings of access to healthcare

As we saw in Chapter 2 there are multiple meanings of "access" but, in general, access encompasses both service provision and service utilization. It is a function of how and where healthcare is provided, dependent upon structural properties of healthcare systems, and on ability to use such services. To that end, the structurationist perspective referred to earlier is singularly appropriate.

A key theme of this book has been to examine the settings within which healthcare takes place. In the most part these are fixed locations, to which people have to travel to access care, but from such places care can be delivered to people in their homes. Regardless, distances have to be overcome, which may be straightforward for some but extremely challenging for others. The stories told in Chapter 1 illustrate this very clearly. In some cases, we have seen imaginative examples of healthcare delivery, as when it is provided by boats to those living on riverbanks in sparsely populated areas. In other situations, care is accessed not at places on the ground but rather in digital space. For those fleeing war-torn areas, or moving across borders to escape the consequences of climate change, accessing healthcare is extremely challenging. The mobilities "turn" in social science is a key perspective in understanding the unequal geographies of healthcare.

Regardless of whether and how healthcare is utilized by the individual, it has consequences for health. If access is impossible, or delayed, health suffers. We saw examples of this when referring to cancer treatment. If there are delays in diagnosis, delays in seeing a specialist for consultation, delays in getting chemotherapy or surgery it is obvious that people living with cancer will bear the consequences. All these delays are, in part at least, shaped by relative location and place, as well as by personal characteristics (such as age, sex, ethnicity). And, of course, by ability to pay, which leads us to the next overarching theme.

Who pays?

There is a moral dimension to accessing healthcare, relating to who pays. Does the responsibility fall mainly on the state, where provision of universal healthcare is a laudable goal? Or should the burden fall more on the individual? Put differently, do we see healthcare as a "right", available to all regardless of ability to pay, or do we see it as a "commodity" for which the market is the appropriate mechanism? While some healthcare systems can be seen as "collectivist" (the UK, Canada, Australia, for example) others are "anti-collectivist"; – the US is the prime example (Gatrell & Elliott 2015: 190).

As we noted earlier in the book, the welfare state has been replaced by neoliberalism as the dominant ideology for healthcare. Such an ideology posits that healthcare is a privilege not a fundamental right. Provision is to be via the private sector with the "consumer" paying out of their pocket rather than relying on the state. Although there are insurance schemes to help defray the cost of treatment these are not always affordable for those on low incomes. We have seen above how there are many people uninsured in the US, and this is patterned socially and geographically. There are inequities.

Issues of equity clearly arise when some who need healthcare can afford to pay for private treatment while others cannot. As we have seen, in the UK's National Health Service there can be long waiting times for surgery (e.g. hip and other joint replacements) but these can be circumvented if the patient is willing to pay for private treatment. This leads us to the overarching theme of the book.

Equity of access

The book's subtitle makes it clear that the focus has been on the "unequal geographies" of healthcare. In terms of spatial accessibility, it is obvious that not everyone can live close to a clinic or hospital; there is "inequality" simply because of population distribution. What matters more is whether some social groups are disadvantaged as a result of relative location. There remains in place the "inverse care law", first outlined by Julian Tudor Hart 55 years ago. Those in need of good healthcare are invariably least likely to have access to it. This applies to many marginalized groups, whether these are minority ethnic or Indigenous populations, those with disabilities or transgender people. It certainly applies to refugees. It also applies to older people and to women in many circumstances, particularly in parts of the Global South. Consequently, these inequities vary from place to place. Even under the collectivist healthcare systems referred to above there are spatial inequities in access. Universal healthcare is no guarantee of equity.

History matters

The rise of neoliberalism since the late 1970s has, in many countries, drastically curtailed state provision for healthcare and promoted instead a free-market agenda to finance it. International financial institutions imposed structural adjustment programmes on many countries in the Global South, while countries in the Global North (the UK and Greece, for example) have seen cutbacks in healthcare under the guise of "austerity". The impact of austerity on healthcare plays out differently in different places and for different social groups.

Healthcare systems are not immutable. When new governments form they invariably put their own stamp on healthcare provision. We have seen this in the US, where the Trump administration has implemented funding cuts for Medicaid, with severe impacts for poor people and those with disabilities. Inevitably, this has consequences for the equity of provision. In the UK the Labour government, elected for a five-year term in 2024, has proposed to "get the NHS back on its feet". A key element in its strategy is to increase the use of digital technologies, whether through new apps for booking appointments and managing prescriptions, or the use of surgical robots. The extent to which this lessens, or even widens, inequities in healthcare access remains to be seen, although an intriguing study in England (Morton *et al.* 2024) suggests that robotic colorectal surgery – despite a relatively small number of cases – is less commonly undertaken for people living in deprived areas, reflecting the geographic distribution of centres performing such surgery. I encourage students of health geography to consider these issues in their own research.

Healthcare systems evolve according to international imperatives and national policy. In many parts of the Global South such configurations have been shaped by histories of colonization and decolonization. For countries in Africa that gained independence in the 1960s, "government healthcare carried the stamp of colonial bureaucracy in its organisation" with a focus on "segregated, urban, hospital-based, curative services, which rarely reached more than 15 per cent of the African population" (Turshen 1999: 15). As Turshen noted, countries like Malawi and Sierra Leone were still spending more than 90 per cent of their health budgets on hospital services. Clearly, this had an impact on geographic access to healthcare – both primary and secondary. Of course, in keeping with a historical perspective it is important to recognize that such sectoral and geographic distributions change over time.

All these broad themes lead me to conclude that studying the unequal (and inequitable) geographies of access to healthcare is a key dimension to the wider study of the geographies of health. Such study is intellectually rewarding but, more importantly, politically, economically and morally necessary.

REFERENCES

Abdiwali, S. *et al.* 2024. "Barriers and facilitators to antenatal care services utilisation in Somaliland: a qualitative study". *BMJ Open*. doi: 10.1136/bmjopen-2024-085073.

Abel, Z. *et al.* 2024. "Access to healthcare services during the COVID-19 pandemic: a cross-sectional analysis of income and user-access across 16 economically diverse countries". *BMC Public Health*. doi: 10.1186/s12889-024-20147-y.

Abler, R., J. Adams & P. Gould 1971. *Spatial Organization: The Geographer's View of the World*. Englewood Cliffs, NJ: Prentice-Hall.

Aday, L. & R. Andersen 1974. "A framework for the study of access to medical care". *Health Services Research* 9(3): 208–20.

Adey. P. *et al.* (eds) 2017. *The Routledge Handbook of Mobilities*: London: Routledge.

Adjerid, A. 2024. "COVID-19 in Palestine". *The Lancet Infectious Diseases* 24. doi: 10.1016/S1473-3099(24)00212-3.

Agénor, M. *et al.* (2024) "Barriers to and opportunities for advancing racial equity in cervical cancer screening in the United States". *BMC Women's Health*. doi: 10.1186/s12905-024-03151-7.

Alexis, O. *et al.* 2006. "Overseas nurses' experiences of equal opportunities in the NHS in England". *Journal of Health Organization and Management* 20. doi: 10.1108/14777260610661529.

Allan, H. *et al.* 2004. "The social reproduction of institutional racism: internationally recruited nurses' experiences of the British health services". *Diversity and Equality in Health and Care* 1(2).

Altare, C. *et al.* 2020. "Health services for women, children and adolescents in conflict affected settings: experience from North and South Kivu, Democratic Republic of Congo". *Conflict and Health*. doi: 10.1186/s13031-020-00265-1.

Alves, R. *et al.* 2023. "Primary health care coverage in Brazil: a dataset from 1998 to 2020". *BMC Research Notes*. doi: 10.1186/s13104-023-06323-0.

Amaral, P. *et al.* 2017. "Spatially balanced provision of health equipment: a cross-sectional study oriented to the identification of challenges to access promotion". *International Journal for Equity in Health 16*: doi: 10.1186/s12939-017-0704-x.

Andersen, R. & J. Newman 1973. "Societal and individual determinants of medical care utilization in the United States". *Milbank Memorial Fund Quarterly: Health and Society* 51(1): 95–124.

Andrews, G. 2014. "Co-creating health's lively, moving frontiers: brief observations on the facets and possibilities of non-representational theory". *Health & Place* 30: 165–70.

Andrews, G. & J. Evans 2008. "Understanding the reproduction of health care: towards geographies in health care work". *Progress in Human Geography* 32: 759–80.

Anon 2024. "Equity of access to healthcare for a patient with a severe intellectual disability". *BMJ Evidence-Based Medicine*. doi: 10.1136/bmjebm-2024-112866.

Arnaouti, M. *et al.* 2022. "Medical disaster response: a critical analysis of the 2010 Haiti earthquake". *Frontiers in Public Health*. doi: 10.3389/fpubh.2022.995595.

Asaria, M. *et al.* 2016. "Unequal socioeconomic distribution of the primary care workforce: whole-population small area longitudinal study". *BMJ Open*. doi: 10.1136/bmjopen-2015-008783.

Ashworth, M. *et al.* 2021. "Primary care funding entrenches health inequalities: time for a rethink". *British Journal of General Practice*. doi: 10.3399/bjgp21X714965.
Askew, D. *et al.* 2023. "The Mobile Outreach Boomerang van: taking care to the community". *Medical Journal of Australia*. doi: 10.5694/mja2.51816.
Baatz, R. *et al.* 2022. "Cross-border strategies for access to healthcare in violent conflict: a scoping review". *Journal of Migration and Health*. doi: 10.1016/j.jmh.2022.100093.
Bach-Mortensen, A. *et al.* 2024. "Does outsourcing enable the survival of good care homes? A longitudinal analysis of all care homes in England, 2011–2023". *BMJ Public Health*. doi: 10.1136/bmjph-2024-001227.
Bach-Mortensen, A. *et al.* 2025. "England's two tier care system deepens social care inequalities". *British Medical Journal*. doi: 10.1136/bmj-2025-084808.
Baggott, R. 2004. *Health and Healthcare in Britain*. London: Palgrave Macmillan.
Bahri, C. 2024. "Medical tourism facilitators walk a tightrope between ethics and business". *British Medical Journal*. doi: 10.1136/bmj.q664.
Bar-Haim, S. *et al.* 2023. "The shadows of waiting and care: on discourses of waiting in the history of the British National Health Service". *Wellcome Open Research*. doi: 10.12688/wellcomeopenres.18913.1.
Barr, R. *et al.* 2023. "The international scandal of defective asparaginase: a blight on children with cancer". *Pediatric Blood & Cancer*. doi: 10.1002/pbc.30403.
Basij-Rasikh, M. *et al.* 2024. "Primary healthcare system and provider responses to the Taliban takeover in Afghanistan". *BMJ Global Health*. doi: 10.1136/bmjgh-2023-013760.
Bauer, I. 2017. "More harm than good? The questionable ethics of medical volunteering and international student placements". *Tropical Diseases, Travel Medicine and Vaccines*. doi: 10.1186/s40794-017-0048-y.
Bayati, M. *et al.* 2022. "Inequality in the distribution of COVID-19 vaccine: a systematic review". *International Journal for Equity in Health* 21, doi: 10.1186/s12939-022-01729-x.
Bayley, Z. & L. Crowther 2024. "Hospice topophilia and topophobia as experienced by a local population: implications for equity of access". *Health & Place*. doi: 10.1016/j.healthplace.2024.103381.
Beks, H. *et al.* 2020. "Mobile primary health care clinics for Indigenous populations in Australia, Canada, New Zealand and the United States: a systematic scoping review". *International Journal for Equity in Health*. doi: 10.1186/s12939-020-01306-0.
Bell, S. *et al.* 2018. "From therapeutic landscapes to healthy spaces, places and practices: a scoping review". *Social Science & Medicine* 196: 123–30.
Bell, S. *et al.* 2020. "Long-term healthcare provider availability following large-scale hurricanes: a difference-in-differences study". *PLOS One*. doi: 10.1371/journal.pone.0242823.
Belt, R. *et al.* 2024. "Providing healthcare under the threat of gang-violence: a survey of Haitian healthcare providers". *Conflict & Health*. doi: 10.1186/s13031-024-00612-6.
Benbow, D. 2023. "Commentary: the boy who cried wolf or Cassandra? A consideration of the correct characterization of critics of neoliberal reforms to the English NHS". *International Journal of Social Determinants of Health and Health Service*. doi: 10.1177/27551938221148370.
Beresford, J. & S. Sodero 2025. "Green borders? Challenging paradoxical NHS agendas". In L. Follis *et al.* (eds), *Migrant and Refugee Access to Health Systems*, 197–209. Cheltenham: Elgar.
Biglin, J. 2021. "Photovoice accounts of third places: refugee and asylum seeker populations' experiences of therapeutic space". *Health & Place* 71: doi: 10.1016/j.healthplace.2021.102663.
Bojorquez, I. *et al.* 2024. "Cross-border use of health services: an exploratory mixed-methods project at the Mexico-Guatemala border". *PLOS Global Public Health*. doi: 10.1371/journal.pgph.0003685.
Bonal, M. *et al.* 2024. "A French classification to describe medical deserts: a multi-professional approach based on the first contact with the healthcare system". *International Journal of Health Geographics*. doi: 10.1186/s12942-024-00366-7.
Booth, C. *et al.* 2023. "Common sense oncology: outcomes that matter". *Lancet Oncology*. doi: 10.1016/S1470-2045(23)00319-4.
Borah, L. *et al.* 2023. "State restrictions and geographic access to gender-affirming care for transgender youth". *Journal of the American Medical Association*. doi: 10.1001/jama.2023.11299.
Boyle, M. 2021. *Human Geography: An Essential Introduction*. Chichester: John Wiley.

Bragg, M. *et al.* 2012. "No child or mother left behind: implications for the US from Cuba's maternity homes". *Health Promotion Perspectives* 2. doi: 10.5681/hpp.2012.002.

Brassolotto, J. & T. Daly 2016. "Domesticating dialysis: a feminist political economy analysis of informal renal care in rural British Columbia". *The Canadian Geographer* 60: 519–29.

Brennan, R. & M. Sheraz 2024. "The international community is failing to protect healthcare in armed conflict". *British Medical Journal.* doi: 10.1136/bmj.q2474.

Brown, T. *et al.* 2010. *A Companion to Health and Medical Geography.* Chichester: Wiley-Blackwell.

Brown, T. *et al.* 2018. *Health Geographies: A Critical Introduction.* Chichester: Wiley-Blackwell.

Burnett, K. *et al.* 2020. "Indigenous Peoples, settler colonialism, and access to health care in rural and northern Ontario". *Health & Place* 66. doi: 10.1016/j.healthplace.2020.102445.

Burns, A. *et al.* 2023. "The maternal health of American Indian and Alaska Native people: a scoping review". *Social Science & Medicine.* doi: 10.1016/j.socscimed.2022.115584.

Büyüm, A. *et al.* 2020. "Decolonising global health: if not now, when?" *BMJ Global Health.* doi: 10.1136/bmjgh-2020-003394.

Cacciatore, J. *et al.* 2020. "Evaluating care farming as a means to care for those in trauma and grief". *Health & Place* 62. doi: 10.1016/j.healthplace.2019.102281.

Caincross, F. 1997. *The Death of Distance.* Boston, MA: Harvard Business School Press.

Carlson, M. *et al.* 2010. "Geographic access to hospice in the United States". *Journal of Palliative Medicine.* doi: 10.1089/jpm.2010.0209.

Carr, B. *et al.* 2017. "Disparities in access to trauma care in the United States: a population-based analysis". *Injury* 48. doi: 10.1016/j.injury.2017.01.008.

Carrillo, J. *et al.* 2011. "Defining and targeting health care access barriers". *Journal of Health Care for the Poor and Underserved* 22(2): 562–75.

Castleden, H. *et al.* 2010. '"It's not necessarily the distance on the map...': using place as an analytic tool to elucidate geographic issues central to rural palliative care". *Health & Place* 16. doi: 10.1016/j.healthplace.2009.10.011.

Castellano, T. *et al.* 2022. "Cervical cancer geographical burden analyzer: An interactive, open-access tool for understanding geographical disease burden in patients with recurrent or metastatic cervical cancer". *Gynecologic Oncology.* doi: 10.1016/j.ygyno.2022.12.004.

Castro, M. *et al.* 2019. "Brazil's unified health system: the first 30 years and prospects for the future". *Lancet* 394. doi: 10.1016/S0140-6736(19)31243-7.

Chekar, C. *et al.* 2024. "Gender, flexibility and workforce in the NHS: a qualitative study". *International Journal of Health Planning & Management* 39. doi: 10.1002/hpm.3784.

Chen, L. *et al.* 2023. "Spatial accessibility evaluation and location optimization of primary healthcare in China: a case study of Shenzhen". *Geohealth.* doi: 10.1029/2022GH000753.

Chen, T. & J. Pan 2022. "The effect of spatial access to primary care on potentially avoidable hospitalizations of the elderly: evidence from Chishui City, China". *Social Indicators Research* 160. doi: 10.1007/s11205-020-02413-9.

Chevillard, G. *et al.* 2018. "Medical deserts in France: Current state of research and future trends". *L'Espace géographique* 1–19. [English translation at https://shs.cairn.info/journal-espace-geographique-2018-4-page-362?lang=en].

Chomsky, N. 2011. "The state-corporate complex: a threat to freedom and survival", talk given by Noam Chomsky at University of Toronto, 7 April 2011. https://chomsky.info/20110407-2/.

Christiansen, I. 2017. "Commodification of healthcare and its consequences". *World Review of Political Economy* 8: 82–103.

Chukwusa, E. *et al.* 2020. "Regional variations in geographic access to inpatient hospices and place of death: a population based study in England, UK". *PLOS One.* doi: 10.1371/journal.pone.0231666.

Collyer, F. *et al.* 2017. "Gatekeepers in the healthcare sector: knowledge and Bourdieu's concept of field". *Social Science & Medicine* 186: 96–103.

Connell, J. 2011. "A new inequality? Privatisation, urban bias, migration and medical tourism". *Asia Pacific Viewpoint.* doi: 10.1111/j.1467-8373.2011.01454.x.

Connell, J. & M. Walton-Roberts 2016. "What about the workers? The missing geographies of health care". *Progress in Human Geography.* doi: 10.1177/0309132515570513.

Conradson, D. 2003. "Geographies of care: spaces, practices, experiences". *Social & Cultural Geography* 4(4). doi: 10.1080/1464936032000137894.
Costa-Font, J. & A. Rico 2006. "Devolution and the interregional inequalities in health and healthcare in Spain". *Regional Studies*. doi: 10.1080/00343400600984346.
Cresswell, T. 2006. *On the Move: Mobility in the Modern Western World*. Abingdon: Routledge.
Cresswell, T. 2024. *Geographic Thought: A Critical Introduction*. Second edition. Chichester: Wiley-Blackwell.
Criel, B. *et al.* 2020. "Can mutual health organisations influence the quality and the affordability of healthcare provision? The case of the Democratic Republic of Congo". *PLOS One*. doi: 10.1371/journal.pone.0231660.
Cromley, E. & S. McLafferty 2011. *GIS and Public Health*. Second edition. New York: Guilford Press.
Curtis, S. 2004. *Health and Inequality: Geographical Perspectives*. London: Sage.
Cutchin, M. 2007. "Therapeutic landscapes for older people: care with commodification, liminality, and ambiguity". In A. Williams (ed.), *Therapeutic Landscapes*, 181–98. Aldershot: Ashgate.
Daca, C. *et al.* 2020. "Socio-economic and demographic factors associated with reproductive and child health preventive care in Mozambique: a cross-sectional study". *International Journal for Equity in Health* 19. doi: 10.1186/s12939-020-01303-3.
Davy, C. *et al.* 2016. "Access to primary health care services for Indigenous peoples: a framework synthesis". *International Journal for Equity in Health*. doi: 10.1186/s12939-016-0450-5.
de Andrade, L. *et al.* 2022. "Impact of socioeconomic factors and health determinants on preterm birth in Brazil: a register-based study". *BMC Pregnancy and Childbirth*. doi: 10.1186/s12884-022-05201-0.
de Oliveira, A. *et al.* 2017. "Challenges for ensuring availability and accessibility to health care services under Brazil's Unified Health System (SUS)". *Ciência & Saúde Coletiva* 22: doi: 10.1590/1413-81232017224.31382016.
Diaz, J. *et al.* 2023. "Evaluating rural health disparities in Colombia: identifying barriers and strategies to advancing refugee health". *International Journal of Environmental Research and Public Health*. doi: 10.3390/ijerph20206948.
Doetsch, J. *et al.* 2023. "A scoping review on the impact of austerity on healthcare access in the European Union: rethinking austerity for the most vulnerable". *International Journal for Equity in Health*. doi: 10.1186/s12939-022-01806-1.
Dolby, T. *et al.* 2022. "Monitoring sociodemographic inequality in COVID-19 vaccination uptake in England: a national linked data study". *Journal of Epidemiology and Community Health*. doi: 10.1136/jech-2021-218415.
Dong, W. *et al.* 2022. "Medicaid expansion associated with reduction in geospatial breast cancer stage at diagnosis disparities". *Journal of Public Health Management Practices*. doi: 10.1097/PHH.0000000000001514.
Dorling, D. 2023. *Shattered Nation: Inequality and the Geography of a Failing State*. London: Verso.
dos Anjos Luis, A. & P. Cabral 2016. "Geographic accessibility to primary healthcare centers in Mozambique". *International Journal for Equity in Health* 15. doi: 10.1186/s12939-016-0455-0.
Dubey, S. *et al.* 2023. "Evolution of Government-funded health insurance for universal health coverage in India". *Lancet Regional Health Southeast Asia*. doi: 10.1016/j.lansea.2023.100180.
Durham, J. & S. Blondell 2017. "A realist synthesis of cross-border patient movement from low and middle income countries to similar or higher income countries". *Global Health*. doi: 10.1186/s12992-017-0287-8.
Eaton, J. *et al.* 2023. "The negative impact of global health worker migration, and how it can be addressed". *Public Health* 225. doi: 10.1016/j.puhe.2023.09.014.
Engebretsen, E. & M. Baker 2024. "The rhetoric of decolonizing global health fails to address the reality of settler colonialism: Gaza as a case in point". *International Journal of Health Policy and Management*. doi: 10.34172/ijhpm.2024.8419.
English, J. *et al.* 2008. "Health, healing and recovery: therapeutic landscapes and the everyday lives of breast cancer survivors". *Social Science & Medicine* 67(1): 68–78.
Eni, R. *et al.* 2021. "Decolonizing health in Canada: a Manitoba first nation perspective". *International Journal for Equity in Health*. doi: 10.1186/s12939-021-01539-7.

Everhart, A. *et al.* 2023. "Measuring geographic access to transgender hormone therapy in Texas: a three-step floating catchment area analysis". *Spatial and Spatio-temporal Epidemiology*. doi: 10.1016/j.sste.2023.100585.
Exworthy, M. *et al.* 2023. *The NHS at 75: The State of UK Health Policy*. Bristol: Policy Press.
Fabius, C. *et al.* 2023. "The role of place in person- and family-oriented long-term services and supports". *The Milbank Quarterly*. doi: 10.1111/1468-0009.12664.
Farmer, P. 2020. *Fevers, Feuds, and Diamonds: Ebola and the Ravages of History*. New York: Farrar, Straus & Giroux.
Fernandez, G. & P. Boulle 2013. "Where conflict's medical consequences remain unchanged". *The Lancet* 381. doi: 10.1016/S0140-6736(13)60664-9.
Fiedler, J. 1981. "A review of the literature on access and utilization of medical care with special emphasis on rural primary care". *Social Science & Medicine* 15C: 129–42.
Follis, L. *et al.* (eds) 2025. *Migrant and Refugee Access to Health Systems: Challenging (Im)mobilities in Healthcare*. Cheltenham: Elgar.
Fonseca, B. *et al.* 2021. "Geographic accessibility to cancer treatment in Brazil: a network analysis". *Lancet Regional Health Americas*. doi: 10.1016/j.lana.2021.100153.
Fox, H. *et al.* 2021. "Ethnic, socio-economic and geographic inequities in maternal health service coverage in Australia". *International Journal of Health Planning and Management* 36(6): 2182–98.
Fraser, A. *et al.* 2019. "Biopolitics, space and hospital reconfiguration". *Social Science & Medicine* 230: 111–21.
French, M. *et al.* 2023. "Facilitating equitable access to hospice care in socially deprived areas: a mixed methods multiple case study". *Palliative Medicine* 37. doi: 10.1177/02692163221133977.
Frey, A. *et al.* 2024. "Inequalities in healthcare use during the COVID-19 pandemic". *Nature Communications*. doi: 10.1038/s41467-024-45720-2.
Frydman, J. *et al.* 2022. "Telemedicine utilization in the ambulatory palliative care setting: are there disparities?" *Journal of Pain and Symptom Management*. doi: 10.1016/j.jpainsymman.2021.09.019.
Garcia-Saiso, S. *et al.* 2024. "Artificial intelligence as a potential catalyst to a more equitable cancer care". *JMIR Cancer*. doi: 10.2196/57276.
Garnelo, L. *et al.* 2020. "Barriers to access and organization of primary health care services for rural riverside populations in the Amazon". *International Journal for Equity in Health 19*. doi: 10.1186/s12939-020-01171-x.
Gatrell, A. 2011. *Mobilities and Health*. Farnham: Ashgate.
Gatrell, A. 2023. *Global Health: Geographical Connections*. Newcastle upon Tyne: Agenda Publishing.
Gatrell, A. & S. Elliott 2015. *Geographies of Health: An Introduction*. Chichester: John Wiley & Sons.
Gatrell, A. & D. Wood 2012. "Variation in geographic access to specialist inpatient hospices in England and Wales". *Health & Place* 18. doi: 10.1016/j.healthplace.2012.03.009.
Gatwiri, K. *et al.* 2021. "Black lives matter in healthcare: racism and implications for health inequity among Aboriginal and Torres Strait Islander Peoples in Australia". *International Journal of Environmental Research and Public Health*. doi: 10.3390/ijerph18094399.
Gaughan, J. *et al.* 2015. "Testing the bed-blocking hypothesis: does nursing and care home supply reduce delayed hospital discharges? *Health Economics*. doi: 10.1002/hec.3150.
Geldsetzer, P. *et al.* 2020. "Mapping physical access to health care for older adults in sub-Saharan Africa and implications for the COVID-19 response: a cross-sectional analysis". *Lancet Healthy Longevity*. doi: 10.1016/S2666-7568(20)30010-6.
Gesler, W. 1992. "Therapeutic landscapes: medical issues in light of the new cultural geography". *Social Science & Medicine* 34: 735–46.
Gesler, W. & R. Kearns 2002. *Culture/Place/Health*. London: Routledge.
Girotra, S. *et al.* 2023. "Utilization and determinants of adequate quality antenatal care services in India: evidence from the National Family Health Survey (NFHS-5) (2019-21)". *BMC Pregnancy Childbirth* 23. doi: 10.1186/s12884-023-06117-z.
Glick Schiller, N. & N. Salazar 2013. "Regimes of mobility across the world". *Journal of Ethnic and Migration Studies* 39: 183–200.

Gligorić, K. *et al.* 2023. "Revealed versus potential spatial accessibility of healthcare and changing patterns during the COVID-19 pandemic". *Communications Medicine*. doi: 10.1038/s43856-023-00384-9.
Gogoi, N. & S. Sumesh 2022. "The political economy of public health inequalities and inequities in India: complexities, challenges, and strategies for inclusive public health care policy". *International Journal of Health Services* 52(2): 225–35.
Gomes, R. *et al.* 2024. "Therapeutic itineraries in health care in Quilombola communities". *Ciencia & Saude Coletiva*. doi: 10.1590/1413-81232024293.01602023.
Gómez-Dantés, O. 2018. "Cuba's health system: hardly an example to follow". *Health Policy and Planning*. doi: 10.1093/heapol/czy035.
Good, C. 1977. "Traditional medicine: an agenda for medical geography". *Social Science & Medicine*. doi: 10.1016/0037-7856(77)90156-1.
Goodair, B. & A. Reeves 2022. "Outsourcing health-care services to the private sector and treatable mortality rates in England, 2013–20: an observational study of NHS privatisation". *Lancet Public Health* 7. doi: 10.1016/S2468-2667(22)00133-5.
Goodair, B. & A. Reeves 2024. "The effect of health-care privatisation on the quality of care". *Lancet Public Health* 9. doi: 10.1016/S2468-2667(24)00003-3.
Gopfert, A. *et al.* 2021. "Primary care consultation length by deprivation and multimorbidity in England: an observational study using electronic patient records". *British Journal of General Practice* 71. doi: 10.3399/bjgp20X714029.
Göttems, L. & M. Mollo 2020. "Neoliberalism in Latin America: effects on health system reforms". *Revista de Saude Publica*. doi: 10.11606/s1518-8787.2020054001806.
Gould, P. & R. White 1974. *Mental Maps*. London: Penguin.
Graham, R. & B. Masters-Awatere 2020. "Experiences of Māori of Aotearoa New Zealand's public health system: a systematic review of two decades of published qualitative research". *Australian and New Zealand Journal of Public Health* 44(3): 193–200.
Gréaux, M. *et al.* 2023. "Health equity for persons with disabilities: a global scoping review on barriers and interventions in healthcare services". *International Journal for Equity in Health*. doi: 10.1186/s12939-023-02035-w.
Guagliardo, M. 2004. "Spatial accessibility of primary care: concepts, methods and challenges". *International Journal of Health Geographics* 3. doi: 10.1186/1476-072X-3-3.
Gulliford, M. *et al.* 2002. "What does 'access to health care' mean?" *Journal of Health Services Research and Policy* 7(3): 186–8.
Hendl, T. & A. Shukla 2024. "Can digital health democratize health care?" *Bioethics*. doi: 10.1111/bioe.13266.
Herlitz, S. *et al.* 2023. "Socioeconomic status is associated with process times in the emergency department for patients with chest pain". *Journal of the American College of Emergency Physicians Open*. doi: 10.1002/emp2.13005.
Herrera, C. *et al.* 2024. "Navigating the divide: inequalities in household experiences of healthcare disruption in Latin American and the Caribbean countries amidst COVID-19". *International Journal for Equity in Health*. doi: 10.1186/s12939-024-02337-7.
Herrick, C. 2023. "The 'health workforce crisis' and 'the medical manpower problem': new term, old problems". *Health & Place*. doi: 10.1016/j.healthplace.2023.103132.
Herrick, C. & A. Brooks 2019. "Global health volunteering, the Ebola outbreak, and instrumental humanitarianisms in Sierra Leone". *Transactions, Institute of British Geographers*. doi: 10.1111/tran.12356.
Herrick, C. *et al.* 2022. "Humanitarian inversions: COVID-19 as crisis". *Transactions of the Institute of British Geographers* 47. doi: 10.1111/tran.12544.
Hertz, J. *et al.* 2019. "The distribution of cardiac diagnostic testing for acute coronary syndrome in the Brazilian healthcare system: a national geospatial evaluation of health access". *PLOS One*. doi: 10.1371/journal.pone.0210502.
Hill, P. *et al.* 2014. "The 'empty void' is a crowded space: health service provision at the margins of fragile and conflict affected states". *Conflict & Health*. doi: 10.1186/1752-1505-8-20.
Hinde, S. *et al.* 2021. "Delayed transfers of care for older people: a wider perspective". *Age and Ageing*. doi: 10.1093/ageing/afab035.

Hirose, N. *et al.* 2022. "Universal health coverage of five essential health services in mothers before and after the Haiti 2010 earthquake: a retrospective cohort study using difference-in-difference". *BMC Health Services Research.* doi: 10.1186/s12913-022-08896-1.

Hirt, J. *et al.* 2022. "Staff-to-resident abuse in nursing homes: a scoping review". *BMC Geriatrics.* doi: 10.1186/s12877-022-03243-9.

Hjort, M. *et al.* 2023. "The importance of the outdoor environment for the recovery of psychiatric patients: a scoping review". *International Journal of Environmental Research and Public Health.* doi: 10.3390/ijerph20032240.

Holland, M. 2022. "More than chores: the invisible health work of family caregivers in rural New Brunswick, Canada". *Health & Place.* doi: 10.1016/j.healthplace.2021.102726.

Homedes, N. & A. Ugalde 2005. "Why neoliberal health reforms have failed in Latin America". *Health Policy.* doi: 10.1016/j.healthpol.2004.01.011.

Horner-Johnson, W. *et al.* 2015. "Disparities in receipt of breast and cervical cancer screening for rural women age 18 to 64 with disabilities". *Women's Health Issues.* doi: 10.1016/j.whi.2015.02.04.

Horrill, T. *et al.* 2018. "Understanding access to healthcare among Indigenous peoples: a comparative analysis of biomedical and postcolonial perspectives". *Nursing Inquiry.* doi: 10.1111/nin.12237.

Horrill, T. *et al.* 2025. "'There's just such a mismatch': a qualitative exploration of health systems and organizational-level barriers to accessing cancer services among people experiencing structural marginalization". *International Journal for Equity in Health.* doi: 10.1186/s12939-025-02554-8.

Horton, R. 2022. "Offline: The health of the Uyghur people is all of our concern". *The Lancet* 400, 10 September: 798.

Howard, N. & E. Schneider 2022. "COVID-19 vaccination in Palestine/Israel: citizenship, capitalism, and the logic of elimination". *Health and Human Rights* 24(2): 265–79.

Hughto, J. *et al.* 2016. "Geographic and individual differences in healthcare access for U.S. transgender adults: a multilevel analysis". *LGBT Health.* doi: 10.1089/lgbt.2016.0044.

Hwang, A. *et al.* 2024. "Co-creating humanistic AI AgeTech to support dynamic care ecosystems: a preliminary guiding model". *Gerontologist.* doi: 10.1093/geront/gnae093.

Idehen, E. *et al.* 2018. "Disparities in cervical screening participation: a comparison of Russian, Somali and Kurdish immigrants with the general Finnish population". *International Journal for Equity in Health.* doi: 10.1186/s12939-018-0768-2.

Igonoh, A. 2015. "My experience as an Ebola patient". *American Journal of Tropical Medicine & Hygiene* 92. doi: 10.4269/ajtmh.14-0763.

Iosti, P. 2020. "Territorialization of care and proximities in a community-based primary care system: what are the results on access to care and resident satisfaction? A case study from São Paulo". *Health & Place* 66. doi: 10.1016/j.healthplace.2020.102451.

Iwai, Y. *et al.* 2022. "Narrative trajectories of disaster response: ethical preparedness from Katrina to COVID-19". *Medical Humanities.* doi: 10.1136/medhum-2021-012194.

Jalilian, A. *et al.* 2024. "Length of stay and economic sustainability of virtual ward care in a medium-sized hospital of the UK: a retrospective longitudinal study". *BMJ Open.* doi: 10.1136/bmjopen-2023-081378.

James, P. *et al.* 2020. "Providing healthcare to Ebola survivors: a qualitative exploratory investigation of healthcare providers' views and experiences in Sierra Leone". *Global Public Health* 15: 1380–95. doi: 10.1080/17441692.2020.1762105.

Jelin, E. *et al.* 2024. "Factors associated with patients' experience of accessibility to general practice: results from a national survey in Norway". *BMC Health Services Research.* doi: 10.1186/s12913-024-11460-8.

Jennings, L. *et al.* 2015. "Disparities in mobile phone access and maternal health service utilization in Nigeria: a population based survey". *International Journal of Medical Informatics.* doi: 10.1016/j.ijmedinf.2015.01.016.

Jesudason, T. 2024. "COVAX officially closes". *The Lancet Infectious Diseases.* doi: 10.1016/S1473-3099(24)00133-6.

Jia, P. *et al.* 2022. "Inequalities of spatial primary healthcare accessibility in China". *Social Science & Medicine* 314: doi: 10.1016/j.socscimed.2022.115458.

Jo, O. *et al.* 2021. "Public transport access to NHS dental care in Great Britain". *British Dental Journal.* doi: 10.1038/s41415-021-3002-3.

Jones, B. *et al.* 2023. "Geographic opportunities for assisted reproduction: a study of regional variations in access to fertility treatment in England". *Human Fertility*. doi: 10.1080/14647273.2023.2190040.
Jörg, R. & L. Haldimann 2023. "MHV3SFCA: A new measure to capture the spatial accessibility of health care systems". *Health & Place* 79. doi: 10.1016/j.healthplace.2023.102974.
Joseph, A. & D. Phillips 1984. *Accessibility and Utilization: Geographical Perspectives on Health Care Delivery*. London: Harper & Row.
Kajaria-Montag, H. *et al.* 2024. "Continuity of care increases physician productivity in primary care". *Management Science*. doi: 10.1287/mnsc.2021.02015.
Kamarulzaman, A. *et al.* 2022. "Plugging the medical brain drain". *The Lancet* 400. doi: 10.1016/S0140-6736(22)02087-6.
Kamradt-Scott, A. 2016. "WHO's to blame? The World Health Organization and the 2014 Ebola outbreak in West Africa". *Third World Quarterly*. doi: 10.1080/01436597.2015.1112232.
Kasper, J. & F. Bajunirwe 2012. "Brain drain in sub-Saharan Africa: contributing factors, potential remedies and the role of academic medical centres". *Archives of Disease in Childhood* 97. doi: 10.1136/archdischild-2012-301900.
Kaufmann, V. *et al.* 2004. "Motility: mobility as capital". *International Journal of Urban and Regional Research* 28(4): 745–56.
Kearns, R. & J. Barnett 2000. "'Happy Meals' in the Starship Enterprise: interpreting a moral geography of health care consumption". *Health & Place* 6(2): 81–93.
Kearns, R. & C. Milligan 2020. "Placing therapeutic landscape as theoretical development in Health & Place". *Health & Place*. doi: 10.1016/j.healthplace.2019.102224.
Kearns, R. *et al.* 2020. "Permeable boundaries? Patient perspectives on space and time in general practice waiting rooms". *Health & Place*. doi: 10.1016/j.healthplace.2020.102347.
Keck, C. & G. Reed 2012. "The curious case of Cuba". *American Journal of Public Health* 102. doi: 10.2105/AJPH.2012.300822.
Keegan, G. *et al.* 2023. "Disparities in breast cancer among patients with disabilities: care gaps, accessibility, and best practices". *Journal of the National Cancer Institute*. doi: 10.1093/jnci/djad130.
Kepper, M. *et al.* 2024. "Expanding a behavioral view on digital health access: drivers and strategies to promote equity". *Journal of Medical Internet Research*. doi: 10.2196/51355.
Kieny, M. *et al.* 2017. "Strengthening health systems for universal health coverage and sustainable development". *Bulletin of the World Health Organization*. doi: 10.2471/BLT.16.187476.
Kim, Y. *et al.* 2018. "Enhancing healthcare accessibility measurements using GIS: a case study in Seoul, Korea". *PLOS One*. doi: 10.1371/journal.pone.0193013.
Kimario, E. *et al.* 2024. "Identifying optimal locations for the development of health facilities towards the attainment of universal health coverage using geospatial techniques in Kishapu district, Tanzania". *Health & Place*. doi: 10.1016/j.healthplace.2024.103369.
Kipp, W. *et al.* 2007. "Family caregivers in rural Uganda: the hidden reality". *Health Care for Women International*. doi: 10.1080/07399330701615275.
Kirkwood, G. *et al.* 2024. "Private sector expansion and the widening NHS treatment gap between rich and poor in England: admissions for NHS-funded elective primary hip and knee replacements between 1997/98 and 2018/19". *Health Policy*. doi: 10.1016/j.healthpol.2024.105118.
Kohli, R. *et al.* 2012. "Caring for caregivers of people living with HIV in the family: a response to the HIV pandemic from two urban slum communities in Pune, India". *PLOS One*. doi: 10.1371/journal.pone.0044989.
Kovacs, R. *et al.* 2021. "Socioeconomic inequalities in the quality of primary care under Brazil's national pay-for-performance programme: a longitudinal study of family health teams". *Lancet Global Health*. doi: 10.1016/S2214-109X(20)30480-0.
Kroelinger, C. *et al.* 2021. "Geographic access to critical care obstetrics for women of reproductive age by race and ethnicity". *American Journal of Obstetrics and Gynecology* 224. doi: 10.1016/j.ajog.2020.08.042.
Kuehn, M. *et al.* 2022. "Assessing barriers to access and equity for COVID-19 vaccination in the US". *BMC Public Health* 22. doi: 10.1186/s12889-022-14636-1.
Kukulka, K. *et al.* 2024. "A qualitative exploration of factors influencing healthcare utilization among rural Missourians: 'we have to be bleeding, broken' ". *Health & Place*. doi: 10.1016/j.healthplace.2024.103367.

Kunyenje, C. *et al.* 2023. "COVID-19 vaccine inequity in African low-income countries". *Frontiers in Public Health*. doi: 10.3389/fpubh.2023.1087662.

Kuper, H. & P. Heydt 2019. *The Missing Billion: Access to Health Services for 1 Billion People With Disabilities*. London: London School of Hygiene and Tropical Medicine. https://www.lshtm.ac.uk/TheMissingBillion.

Kvæl, L. & H. Gautun 2023. "Social inequality in navigating the healthcare maze: care trajectories from hospital to home via intermediate care for older people in Norway". *Social Science & Medicine*. doi: 10.1016/j.socscimed.2023.116142.

Kwiringira, J. *et al.* 2021. "'When will the doctor be around so that I come by?!' Geo-socio effects on health care supply, access and utilisation: experiences from Kalangala Islands, Uganda". *BMC Health Services Research*. doi: 10.1186/s12913-021-07204-7.

Lafaut, D. 2021. "Beyond biopolitics: the importance of the later work of Foucault to understand care practices of healthcare workers caring for undocumented migrants". *BMC Medical Ethics*. doi: 10.1186/s12910-021-00726-z.

Lane, S. *et al.* 2021. "Impacts of the Global Gag Rule on sexual and reproductive health and rights in the Global South: a scoping review". *Global Public Health*. doi: 10.1080/17441692.2020.1840611.

Lavergne, M. *et al.* 2023. "Disparities in access to primary care are growing wider in Canada". *Healthcare Management Forum*. doi: 10.1177/08404704231183599.

Lenguerrand, E. *et al.* 2023. "Inequalities in provision of hip and knee replacement surgery for osteoarthritis by age, sex, and social deprivation in England between 2007–2017: a population-based cohort study of the National Joint Registry". *PLOS Medicine*. doi: 10.1371/journal.pmed.1004210.

Levesque, J.-F. *et al.* 2013. "Patient-centred access to health care: conceptualising access at the interface of health systems and populations". *International Journal for Equity in Health* 12. doi: 10.1186/1475-9276-12-18.

Lilley, R. 2019. "Geographical and population disparities in timely access to prehospital and advanced level emergency care in New Zealand: a cross-sectional study". *BMJ Open*. doi: 10.1136/bmjopen-2018-026026.

Limaye, N. *et al.* 2018. "The Amazon Hope: a qualitative and quantitative assessment of a mobile clinic ship in the Peruvian Amazon". *PLOS One*. doi: 10.1371/journal.pone.0196988.

Lin, J. *et al.* 2023. "The action logic of the older adults about health-seeking in south rural China". *BMC Public Health* 23: doi: 10.1186/s12889-023-17314-y.

Lincoln, A. *et al.* 2023. "Global report on COVID-19 vaccination and reasons not to vaccinate among adults with intellectual disabilities: results from secondary analyses of Special Olympics' program planning". *PLOS Global Public Health*. doi: 10.1371/journal.pgph.0001367.

Llop-Gironés, A. *et al.* 2019 "Inequalities in the access to and quality of healthcare in Mozambique: evidence from the household budget survey". *International Journal for Quality in Health Care* 31(8): 577–82.

Lopes, C. *et al.* 2016. "Inequities in access to depression treatment: results of the Brazilian National Health Survey – PNS". *International Journal for Equity in Health*. doi: 10.1186/s12939-016-0446-1.

Lu, L. & J. Zeng 2018. "Inequalities in the geographic distribution of hospital beds and doctors in traditional Chinese medicine from 2004 to 2014". *International Journal for Equity in Health*. doi: 10.1186/s12939-018-0882-1.

Ludwick, A. *et al.* 2009. "Distances to emergency department and to primary care provider's office affect emergency department use in children". *Academic Emergency Medicine* 16. doi: 10.1111/j.1553-2712.2009.00395.x.

Luo, W. & F. Wang 2003. "Measures of spatial accessibility to healthcare in a GIS environment: synthesis and a case study in Chicago region". *Environment & Planning B* 30(6): 865–84.

Machado, C. & G. Silva 2019. "Political struggles for a universal health system in Brazil: successes and limits in the reduction of inequalities". *Globalization & Health* 15. doi: 10.1186/s12992-019-0523-5.

Maddock, J. *et al.* 2022. "Inequalities in healthcare disruptions during the COVID-19 pandemic: evidence from 12 UK population-based longitudinal studies". *BMJ Open*. doi: 10.1136/ bmjopen-2022-064981.

Magadi, J. & M. Magadi 2022. "Ethnic inequalities in patient satisfaction with primary health care in England: evidence from recent General Practitioner Patient Surveys (GPPS)". *PLOS ONE*. doi: 10.1371/journal.pone.0270775.

Mai, S. *et al.* 2022. "Factors associated with access to healthcare services for older adults with limited activities of daily living". *Frontiers in Public Health*. doi: 10.3389/fpubh.2022.921980.

Maini, R. *et al.* 2014. "Picking up the bill – improving health-care utilisation in the Democratic Republic of Congo through user fee subsidisation: a before and after study". *BMC Health Services Research* 14. doi: 10.1186/s12913-014-0504-6.

Malatzky, C. *et al.* 2020. "The utility of conceptualisations of place and belonging in workforce retention: a proposal for future rural health research". *Health & Place* 62. doi: 10.1016/j.healthplace.2019.102279.

Malone, N. *et al.* 2020. "Mobile health clinics in the United States". *International Journal for Equity in Health*. doi: 10.1186/s12939-020-1135-7.

Marmot, M. 2018. "An inverse care law for our time". *British Medical Journal*. doi: 10.1136/bmj.k3216.

Martin, D. & J. Roe 2022. "Enabling care: Maggie's centres and the affordance of hope". *Health & Place* 78. doi: 10.1016/j.healthplace.2022.102758.

Martins, H. 2024. "Left behind places in Brazil: the dynamics of regional inequalities and public policies in the early 21st century". *Cambridge Journal of Regions, Economy and Society* 17: 235–48.

Mavodza, C. *et al.* 2019. "The impacts of the global gag rule on global health: a scoping review. *Global Health Research and Policy*. doi: 10.1186/s41256-019-0113-3.

McFadden, A. *et al.* 2018. "Gypsy, Roma and Traveller access to and engagement with health services: a systematic review". *European Journal of Public Health*. doi: 10.1093/eurpub/ckx226.

McGee-Avila, J. *et al.* 2023. "Disparities in geospatial patterns of cancer care within urban counties and structural inequities in access to oncology care". *Health Services Research*. doi: 10.1111/1475-6773.14182.

Meghani, Z. 2013. "The ethics of medical tourism: from the United Kingdom to India seeking medical care". *International Journal of Health Services Research*. doi: 10.2190/HS.43.4.k.

Miller, E. *et al.* 2022. "Racial disparities in access to public green spaces: using Geographic Information Systems to identify underserved populations in a small American city". *Environmental Justice* 15. doi: 10.1089/env.2021.0067.

Miller, R. *et al.* 2021. "When technology precedes regulation: the challenges and opportunities of e-pharmacy in low-income and middle-income countries". *BMJ Global Health*. doi: 10.1136/bmjgh-2021-005405.

Milligan, C. & A. Bingley 2007. "Restorative places or scary spaces? The impact of woodland on the mental well-being of young adults". *Health & Place* 13(4): 799–811.

Milligan, C. & J. Wiles 2010. "Landscapes of care". *Progress in Human Geography* 34(6): 736–54.

Milligan, C. *et al.* 2011. "Telecare and older people: who cares where?" *Social Science & Medicine*. doi: 10.1016/j.socscimed.2010.08.014.

Moore, A. *et al.* 2013. "'I am closer to this place': space, place and notions of home in lived experiences of hospice day care". *Health & Place*. doi: 10.1016/j.healthplace.2012.11.002.

Moosa, S. *et al.* 2014. "The inverse primary care law in sub-Saharan Africa: a qualitative study of the views of migrant health workers". *British Journal of General Practice*. doi: 10.3399/bjgp14X680089.

Mor, V. *et al.* 2004. "Driven to tiers: socioeconomic and racial disparities in the quality of nursing home care". *The Milbank Quarterly*. doi: 10.1111/j.0887-378X.2004.00309.x.

Morgan, R. *et al.* 2022. "Women healthcare workers' experiences during COVID-19 and other crises: a scoping review". *International Journal of Nursing Studies Advances*. doi: 10.1016/j.ijnsa.2022.100066.

Morton, A. *et al.* 2024. "Regional variations and deprivation are linked to poorer access to laparoscopic and robotic colorectal surgery: a national study in England". *Techniques in Coloproctology*. doi: 10.1007/s10151-023-02874-3.

Mpofu, C. *et al.* 2016. "The ethics of medical practitioner migration from low-resourced countries to the developed world: a call for action by health systems and individual doctors". *Bioethical Inquiry* 13. doi: 10.1007/s11673-016-9726-0.

Mukendi, D. *et al.* 2019. "Distribution and quality of emergency obstetric care service delivery in the Democratic Republic of the Congo: it is time to improve regulatory mechanisms". *Reproductive Health* 16. doi: 10.1186/s12978-019-0772-z.

Mulyanto, J. *et al.* 2019. "Geographical inequalities in healthcare utilisation and the contribution of compositional factors: a multilevel analysis of 497 districts in Indonesia". *Health & Place*. doi: 10.1016/j.healthplace.2019.102236.

Nakayama, L. *et al.* 2023. "The digital divide in Brazil and barriers to telehealth and equal digital health care: analysis of internet access using publicly available data". *Journal of Medical Internet Research*. doi: 10.2196/42483.
Nandi, S. *et al.* 2018. "Assessing geographical inequity in availability of hospital services under the state-funded universal health insurance scheme in Chhattisgarh state, India, using a composite vulnerability index". *Global Health Action*. doi: 10.1080/16549716.2018.1541220.
Nanyonjo, A. *et al.* 2023. "Community efforts to promote vaccine uptake in a rural setting: a qualitative interview study". *Health Promotion International*. doi: 10.1093/heapro/daad088.
NaRanong, A. & V. NaRanong 2011. "The effects of medical tourism: Thailand's experience". *Bulletin of the World Health Organization*. doi: 10.2471/BLT.09.072249.
Naser-Najjab, N. 2024. *COVID-19 in Palestine: The Settler Colonial Context*. London: Bloomsbury.
Nie, P. *et al.* 2020. "Socioeconomic position and the health gradient in Cuba: dimensions and mechanisms". *BMC Public Health*. doi: 10.1186/s12889-020-08980-3.
Nkosi, M. 2023. "Patients' experiences in the use of mobile health clinics in KwaMachi rural area of KwaZulu-Natal, South Africa". *Dialogues in Health*. doi: 10.1016/j.dialog.2023.100164.
Nogueira, M. *et al.* 2019. "Inequities in access to mammographic screening in Brazil". *Cadernos de Saúde Pública*. doi: 10.1590/0102-311X00099817.
Nordling, L. 2019. "A fairer way forward for AI in health care". *Nature*. doi: 10.1038/d41586-019-02872-2.
Nyamugira, A. *et al.* 2022. "Towards the achievement of universal health coverage in the Democratic Republic of Congo: does the country walk its talk?" *BMC Health Services Research* 22. doi: 10.1186/s12913-022-08228-3.
Nyando, M. *et al.* 2023. "Perceptions of pregnant women on antenatal care visit during their first trimester at area 25 health center in Lilongwe, Malawi: a qualitative study". *BMC Women's Health*. doi: 10.1186/s12905-023-02800-7.
Obrist, B. *et al.* 2007. "Access to health care in contexts of livelihood insecurity: a framework for analysis and action". *PLOS Medicine*. doi: 10.1371/journal.pmed.0040308.
Obrochta, C. *et al.* 2022. "The impact of patient travel time on disparities in treatment for early stage lung cancer in California". *PLOS One* 17. doi: 10.1371/journal.pone.0272076.
Ormond, M. & D. Sulianti 2014. "More than medical tourism: lessons from Indonesia and Malaysia on South–South intra-regional medical travel". *Current Issues in Tourism* 20. doi: 10.1080/13683500.2014.937324.
Ortega, F. & A. Pele 2023. "Brazil's unified health system: 35 years and future challenges". *Lancet Regional Health – Americas* 28. doi: 10.1016/j.lana.2023.100631.
Osei, M. *et al.* 2023. "Persistence of unequal access to classical hematology: telemedicine visits by race and other demographics during the COVID-19 pandemic". *Telemedicine Journal and e-Health*. doi: 10.1089/tmj.2022.0505.
Paccoud, I. *et al.* 2020. "A Bourdieusian approach to class-related inequalities: the role of capitals and capital structure in the utilisation of healthcare services in later life". *Sociology of Health and Illness* 42(3): 510–25.
Padmaja, M. & D. Behera 2023. "Disruptions in accessing women's health care services: evidence using COVID-19 Health Services Disruption Survey". *Maternal & Child Health Journal*. doi: 10.1007/s10995-022-03585-1.
Parr, H. 2003. "Medical geography: care and caring". *Progress in Human Geography* 27(2): 212–21.
Patel, J. *et al.* 2024. "Reshaping the equitable and inclusive access to healthcare: a qualitative study". *Clinical Epidemiology and Global Health*. doi: 10.1016/j.cegh.2024.101544.
Patil, D. *et al.* 2023. "Unpacking the role of transport inequalities among older adults for accessing healthcare in Bengaluru, India". *Global Public Health*. doi: 10.1080/17441692.2023.2274438.
Patwardhan, B. *et al.* 2023. "Evidence-based traditional medicine for transforming global health and well-being". *Complementary Therapies in Medicine*. doi: 10.1016/j.ctim.2023.102970.
Penchansky, R. & J. Thomas 1981. "The concept of access". *Medical Care* 19(2): 127–40.
Peroni, F. *et al.* 2019. "Realizing the right to health in Brazil's Unified Health System through the lens of breast and cervical cancer". *International Journal for Equity in Health* 18. doi: 10.1186/s12939-019-0938-x.

Perry, T. & A. Bernasek 2024. "Profits over care? An analysis of the relationship between corporate capitalism in the healthcare industry and cancer mortality in the United States". *Social Science & Medicine*. doi: 10.1016/j.socscimed.2024.116851.

Petricola, S. *et al.* 2022. "Assessing road criticality and loss of healthcare accessibility during floods: the case of Cyclone Idai, Mozambique 2019". *International Journal of Health Geographics* 21. doi: 10.1186/s12942-022-00315-2.

Pfeiffer, J. & R. Chapman 2019. "NGOs, austerity, and universal health coverage in Mozambique". *Globalization and Health* 15. doi: 10.1186/s12992-019-0520-8.

Phillips, D. 1990. *Health and Health Care in the Third World*. Harlow: Longman.

Phillips-Beck, W. *et al.* 2020. "Confronting racism within the Canadian healthcare system: systemic exclusion of First Nations from quality and consistent care". *International Journal of Environmental Research & Public Health*. doi: 10.3390/ijerph17228343.

Porter, S. 2013. "Capitalism, the state and health care in the age of austerity: a Marxist analysis". *Nursing Philosophy* 14(1): 5–16.

Powell, M. 1995. "On the outside looking in: medical geography, medical geographers and access to healthcare". *Health & Place* 1(1): 41–50.

Power, A. 2018. "Spaces of care". In T. Brown *et al.* (eds), *Health Geographies: A Critical Introduction*, 95–113. Chichester: Wiley-Blackwell.

Power, A. & E. Hall 2017. "Placing care in times of austerity". *Social & Cultural Geography*. doi: 10.1080/14649365.2017.1327612.

Privor-Dumm, L. *et al.* 2023. "Vaccine access, equity and justice: COVID-19 vaccines and vaccination". *BMJ Global Health* 8. doi: 10.1136/bmjgh-2023-011881.

Pu, Q. *et al.* 2020. "Improving the spatial accessibility of healthcare in North Kivu, Democratic Republic of Congo". *Applied Geography* 121. doi: 10.1016/j.apgeog.2020.102262.

Punton, G. *et al.* 2022. "'You're on the waiting list': an interpretive phenomenological analysis of young adults' experiences of waiting lists within mental health services in the UK". *PLOS One*. doi: 10.1371/journal.pone.0265542.

Puyvallée, A. & K. Storeng 2022. "COVAX, vaccine donations and the politics of global vaccine inequity". *Globalization and Health*. doi: 10.1186/s12992-022-00801-z.

Qandil, M. 2024. "Gaza: providing emergency care under fire". *Emergency Medicine Journal* 41. doi: 10.1136/emermed-2024-213963.

Qin, A. *et al.* 2024. "Does unequal economic development contribute to the inequitable distribution of healthcare resources? Evidence from China spanning 2001–2020". *Globalization and Health*. doi: 10.1186/s12992-024-01025-z.

Quinn, S. *et al.* 2023. "Dying at home for people experiencing financial hardship and deprivation: how health and social care professionals recognise and reflect on patients' circumstances". *Palliative Care & Social Practice*. doi: 10.1177/26323524231164162.

Rabiou, L. *et al.* 2024. "Mobile outreach clinics for improving health care services accessibility in vulnerable populations of the Diffa Region in Niger: a descriptive study". *International Journal for Equity in Health*. doi: 10.1186/s12939-024-02322-0.

Ramadan, M. *et al.* 2021. "Access to primary healthcare services in conflict-affected fragile states: a subnational descriptive analysis of educational and wealth disparities in Cameroon, Democratic Republic of Congo, Mali, and Nigeria". *International Journal for Equity in Health*. doi: 10.1186/s12939-021-01595-z.

Ramírez de Arellano, A. 2007. "Patients without borders: the emergence of medical tourism". *International Journal of Health Services Research*. doi: 10.2190/4857-468G-2325-47UU.

Raven, J. *et al.* 2018. "Health workers' experiences of coping with the Ebola epidemic in Sierra Leone's health system: a qualitative study". *BMC Health Services Research*. doi: 10.1186/s12913-018-3072-3.

Redhead, G. & R. Lynch 2024. "The unfairness of place: A cultural history of the UK's 'postcode lottery'". *Health & Place*. doi: 10.1016/j.healthplace.2024.103301.

Reibling, N. *et al.* 2019. "Worlds of healthcare: a healthcare system typology of OECD countries". *Health Policy*. doi: 10.1016/j.healthpol.2019.05.001.

Reid, B. *et al.* 2018. "International Voluntary Health Networks (IVHNs): a social-geographical framework". *Health & Place*. doi: 10.1016/j.healthplace.2017.12.005.

Reid, L. 2021. "Anticipating technology-enabled care at home". *Transactions, Institute of British Geographers*. doi: 10.1111/tran.12476.

Ribot, J. & N. Peluso 2003. "A theory of access". *Rural Sociology*. doi: 10.1111/j.1549-0831.2003.tb00133.x.

Robinson, D. *et al.* 2005. "Waiting times for radiotherapy: variation over time and between cancer networks in southeast England". *British Journal of Cancer*. doi: 10.1038/sj.bjc.6602463.

Rocha, T. *et al.* 2017. "Access to emergency care services: a transversal ecological study about Brazilian emergency health care network". *Public Health* 153: 9–15.

Roderick, P. & A. Pollock 2022. "Dismantling the National Health Service in England". *International Journal of Health Services*. doi: 10.1177/00207314221114540.

Rodrigues, K. *et al.* 2021. "Informal and popular healthcare subsystems in a remote rural municipality in the Brazilian Amazon region". *Rural and Remote Health*. doi: 10.22605/RRH6568.

Rotulo, A. *et al.* 2002. "Fiscal federalism vs fiscal decentralization in healthcare: a conceptual framework". *Hippokratia* 24(3): 107–13.

Ryan-Ndegwa, S. *et al.* 2021. "Assessing demographic access to hip replacement surgery in the United Kingdom: a systematic review". *International Journal for Equity in Health*. doi: 10.1186/s12939-021-01561-9.

Rydland, H. *et al.* 2022. "The radically unequal distribution of COVID-19 vaccinations: a predictable yet avoidable symptom of the fundamental causes of inequality". *Humanities and Social Science Communications*. doi: 10.1057/s41599-022-01073-z.

Sahelie, B. *et al.* "Evaluation of mobile clinics by MSF in pastoralist community in Doolo Zone, Somali region, Ethiopia". *BMC Health Services Research*. doi: 10.1186/s12913-025-12282-y.

Sakellariou, D. & E. Rotarou 2017. "The effects of neoliberal policies on access to healthcare for people with disabilities". *International Journal for Equity in Health*. doi: 10.1186/s12939-017-0699-3.

Salles R. *et al.* 2023. "A comprehensive integrated dataset on Brazilian health facilities: from 2005 to 2021. *BMC Research Notes*. doi: 10.1186/s13104-023-06422-y.

Santangelo, O. *et al.* 2024. "COVID-19 vaccination and public health: addressing global, regional, and within-country inequalities". *Vaccines*. doi: 10.3390/vaccines12080885.

Sapkota, S. *et al.* 2023. "The impact of decentralisation on health systems: a systematic review of reviews". *BMJ Global Health*. doi: 10.1136/ bmjgh-2023-013317.

Sarafian, I. *et al.* 2024. "In the margins of stigma: health inequalities among Bulgarian Roma in a post-COVID-19 UK". *BMJ Global Health*. doi: 10.1136/bmjgh-2024-015686.

Saurman, E. 2016. "Improving access: modifying Penchansky and Thomas's theory of access". *Journal of Health Services Research and Policy* 21(1): 36–9.

Scott, K. *et al.* 2021. "Freedom within a cage: how patriarchal gender norms limit women's use of mobile phones in rural central India". *BMJ Global Health*. doi: 10.1136/ bmjgh-2021-005596.

Seedat, S. & M. Rondon 2021. "Women's wellbeing and the burden of unpaid work". *British Medical Journal* 374: doi: 10.1136/bmj.n1972.

Sheller, M. 2013. "The islanding effect: post-disaster mobility systems and humanitarian logistics in Haiti". *Cultural Geographies* 20. doi: 10.1177/1474474012438828.

Sheller, M. 2018. *Mobility Justice: The Politics of Movement in an Age of Extremes*. London: Verso.

Shi, L. *et al.* 1999. "Income inequality, primary care, and health indicators". *Journal of Family Practice* 48: 275–84.

Shi, L. & B. Starfield 2001. "The effect of primary care physician supply and income inequality on mortality among blacks and whites in US metropolitan areas". *American Journal of Public Health*. doi: 10.2105/ajph.91.8.1246.

Shibli, H. *et al.* 2021. "Perceptions about the accessibility of healthcare services among ethnic minority women: a qualitative study among Arab Bedouins in Israel". *International Journal for Equity in Health* 20. doi: 10.1186/s12939-021-01464-9.

Shipton, L. & L. Vitale 2024. "Artificial intelligence and the politics of avoidance in global health". *Social Science & Medicine*. doi: 10.1016/j.socscimed.2024.117274.

Siegel, M. *et al.* 2016. "Developing a composite index of spatial accessibility across different health care sectors: a German example". *Health Policy*. doi: 10.1016/j.healthpol.2016.01.001.

Simmons, C. *et al.* 2022. "Working conditions in the long-term care sector: a comparative study of migrant and native workers in Austria and Sweden". *Health and Social Care in the Community*. doi: 10.1111/hsc.13657.

Sítima, G. *et al.* 2024. "Equity of access to palliative care: a scoping review". *International Journal for Equity in Health*. doi: 10.1186/s12939-024-02321-1.

Siu, A. *et al.* 2022. "Health equity in Hospital at Home: outcomes for economically disadvantaged and non-disadvantaged patients". *Journal of the American Geriatrics Society*. doi: 10.1111/jgs.17759.

Smith, K. 2012. "The problematization of medical tourism: a critique of neoliberalism". *Developing World Bioethics*. doi: 10.1111/j.1471-8847.2012.00318.x.

Smith, K. 2022. *Medical Tourism and Inequality in India: The Hyper-Commodification of Healthcare*. Lanham, MD: Rowman & Littlefield.

Smith, R. 2015. "Healthcare under siege: geopolitics of medical service provision in the Gaza Strip". *Social Science & Medicine* 146. doi: 10.1016/j.socscimed.2015.10.018.

Snyder, J. & V. Crooks 2012. "New ethical perspectives on medical tourism in the developing world". *Developing World Bioethics*. doi: 10.1111/j.1471-8847.2012.00321.x.

Socha-Dietrich, K. & J.-C. Dumont 2021. "International migration and movement of doctors to and within OECD countries – 2000 to 2018: developments in countries of destination and impact on countries of origin". *OECD Health Working Papers*, No. 126, Paris: OECD Publishing. doi: 10.1787/7ca8643e-en.

Song, C. *et al.* 2024. "Revealing spatiotemporal inequalities, hotspots, and determinants in healthcare resource distribution: insights from hospital beds panel data in 2308 Chinese counties". *BMC Public Health* 24. doi: 10.1186/s12889-024-17950-y.

Sowemimo, A. 2023. *Divided: Racism, Medicine and Why We Need to Decolonise Healthcare*. London: Profile.

Sriram, V. *et al.* 2021. "The impact of colonial-era policies on health workforce regulation in India: lessons for contemporary reform". *Human Resources for Health*. doi: 10.1186/s12960-021-00640-w.

Statz, M. & K. Evers 2020. "Spatial barriers as moral failings: what rural distance can teach us about women's health and medical mistrust". *Health & Place* 64: doi: 10.1016/j.healthplace.2020.102396.

Stoller, N. 2003. "Space, place and movement as aspects of health care in three women's prisons". *Social Science & Medicine* 56(11): 2263–75.

Stone, B. *et al.* 2020. "When it rains, it pours: detecting seasonal patterns in utilization of maternal healthcare in Mozambique using routine data". *BMC Health Services Research* 20. doi: 10.1186/s12913-020-05807-0.

Streeter, R. *et al.* 2020. "The geographic alignment of primary care Health Professional Shortage Areas with markers for social determinants of health". *PLOS One* 15. doi: 10.1371/journal. pone.0231443.

Stuckler, D. *et al.* 2011. "Health care capacity and allocations among South Africa's provinces: infrastructure-inequality traps after the end of apartheid". *American Journal of Public Health*. doi: 10.2105/AJPH.2009.184895.

Stuckler, D. *et al.* 2017. "Austerity and health: the impact in the UK and Europe". *European Journal of Public Health*. doi: 10.1093/eurpub/ckx167.

Symer, M. *et al.* 2019. "Barriers to regionalized surgical care: public perspective survey and geospatial analysis". *Annals of Surgery*. doi: 10.1097/SLA.0000000000002556.

Szwarcwald, C. *et al.* 2021. "Changes in the pattern of health services use in Brazil between 2013 and 2019". *Ciencia & Saude Coletiva*. doi: 10.1590/1413-81232021266.

Takeyama, N. *et al.* 2022. "Health-seeking behaviors in Mozambique: a mini-study of ethnonursing". *International Journal of Environmental Research and Public Health* 19. doi: 10.3390/ijerph19042462.

Taniguchi, H. *et al.* 2021. "Trends and projections of universal health coverage indicators in Iraq, 2000–2030: a national and subnational study". *Social Science & Medicine* 270. doi: 10.1016/j.socscimed.2020.113630.

Tankwanchi, A. *et al.* 2015. "Monitoring sub-Saharan African physician migration and recruitment post-adoption of the WHO code of practice: temporal and geographic patterns in the United States". *PLOS One*. doi: 10.1371/journal.pone.0124734.

Tanou, M. *et al.* 2021. "The effects of geographical accessibility to health facilities on antenatal care and delivery services utilization in Benin: a cross-sectional study". *Reproductive Health.* doi: 10.1186/s12978-021-01249-x.

Tanous, O. *et al.* 2023. "Structural racism and the health of Palestinian citizens of Israel". *Global Public Health* 18. doi: 10.1080/17441692.2023.2214608.

Tao, N. *et al.* 2023. "Healthcare collapse in Afghanistan due to political crises, natural catastrophes, and dearth of international aid post-COVID". *Journal of Global Health.* doi: 10.7189/jogh.13.03003.

Tao, Z. *et al.* 2020. "Hierarchical two-step floating catchment area (2SFCA) method: measuring the spatial accessibility to hierarchical healthcare facilities in Shenzhen, China". *International Journal for Equity in Health* 19. doi: 10.1186/s12939-020-01280-7.

Tenorio, A. *et al.* 2024. "A border health crisis at the United States–Mexico border: an urgent call to action". *The Lancet Regional Health – Americas.* doi: 10.1016/j.lana.2024.100676.

Thakkar, N. *et al.* 2023. "Factors associated with underutilization of antenatal care in India: results from 2019–2021 National Family Health Survey". *PLOS One.* doi: 10.1371/journal.pone.0285454.

Thompson, M. 2021. "The geographies of digital health: digital therapeutic landscapes and mobilities". *Health & Place* 70. doi: 10.1016/j.healthplace.2021.102610.

Tobin, J. *et al.* 2022. "Hospice care access inequalities: a systematic review and narrative synthesis". *BMJ Supportive and Palliative Care* 12. doi: 10.1136/bmjspcare-2020-002719.

Tudor Hart, J. 1971. "The inverse care law". The Lancet 297: 405–12.

Turner, A. *et al.* 2022. "Socioeconomic inequality in access to timely and appropriate care in emergency departments". *Journal of Health Economics* 85. doi: 10.1016/j.jhealeco.2022.102668.

Turner, M. *et al.* 2023. "The impact of travel time to cancer treatment centre on post-diagnosis care and mortality among cancer patients in Scotland". *Health & Place* 84. doi: 10.1016/j.healthplace.2023.103139.

Turshen, M. 1999. *Privatizing Health Services in Africa*. New Brunswick, NJ: Rutgers University Press.

UNICEF 2023. "A female health worker's service despite countless challenges". https://www.unicef.org/afghanistan/stories/female-health-workers-service-despite-countless-challenges.

Urry, J. 2007. *Mobilities.* Cambridge: Polity.

Usher, S. & J. Denis 2022. "Network-building by community actors to develop capacities for coproduction of health services following reforms: a case study". *Health Expectations* 25(5): 2275–86.

Vellakkal, S. *et al.* 2017. "A qualitative study of factors impacting accessing of institutional delivery care in the context of India's cash incentive program". *Social Science & Medicine.* doi: 10.1016/j.socscimed.2017.01.059.

Vissoci, J. *et al.* 2019. "Global initiative for children's surgery. Disparities in surgical care for children across Brazil: use of geospatial analysis". *PLOS One.* doi: 10.1371/journal.pone.0220959.

Waitzkin, H. 2020 "Moving beyond capitalism for our health". *International Journal of Health Services Research* 50: 458–62.

Wang, F. & W. Luo 2005. "Assessing spatial and nonspatial factors for healthcare access: towards an integrated approach to defining health professional shortage areas". *Health & Place* 11: 131–46. doi: 10.1016/j.healthplace.2004.02.003.

Wang, J. *et al.* 2021. "Health care visits during the COVID-19 pandemic: a spatial and temporal analysis of mobile device data". *Health & Place.* doi: 10.1016/j.healthplace.2021.102679.

Wang, X. *et al.* 2018. "Spatial accessibility of primary health care in China: a case study in Sichuan Province". *Social Science & Medicine.* doi: 10.1016/j.socscimed.2018.05.023.

Webster, P. 2011. "Iraq's health system yet to heal from ravages of war". *The Lancet* 378. doi: 10.1016/S0140-6736(11)61399-8.

Węgrzynowska, M. *et al.* 2024. "Ukrainian women's maternity care strategies in Poland after the outbreak of the full-scale war: understanding unequal access to quality care". *Social Science & Medicine.* doi: 10.1016/j.socscimed.2024.117409.

Weiss, D. *et al.* 2020. "Global maps of travel time to healthcare facilities". *Nature Medicine* 26: 1835–8.

Welch, E. 2024. *Why Can't I See My GP?* Cardiff: Calon Press.

White, E. *et al.* 2021. "Front-line nursing home staff experiences during the COVID-19 pandemic". *Journal of the American Medical Directors Association.* doi: 10.1016/j.jamda.2020.11.022.

Wigley, A. *et al.* 2020. "Measuring the availability and geographical accessibility of maternal health services across sub-Saharan Africa". *BMC Medicine*. doi: 10.1186/s12916-020-01707-6.
Wilding, S. *et al.* 2022. "Do reasoned action approach variables mediate relationships between demographics and cervical cancer screening intentions or behaviour? An online study of women from the UK". *Social Science & Medicine* 313. doi: 10.1016/j.socscimed.2022.115354.
Wiles, J. 2003. "Daily geographies of caregivers: mobility, routine, scale". *Social Science & Medicine*. doi: 10.1016/s0277-9536(02)00508-7.
Wilkens, J. *et al.* 2024. "From office to digital primary care services: analysing income-related inequalities in utilization". *International Journal for Equity in Health*. doi: 10.1186/s12939-024-02184-6.
Williams, A. 2002. "Changing geographies of care: employing the concept of therapeutic landscapes as a framework in examining home space". *Social Science & Medicine* 55: 141–54.
Williams, A. (ed.) 2007. *Therapeutic Landscapes*. Aldershot: Ashgate.
Williams, H. *et al.* 2004. "On the quality variation of primary health care services: a test of the 'inverse care law' for general practice". *Environment & Planning A* 36: 701–14.
Williamson, C. *et al.* 2023. "Race, insurance, and sex-based disparities in access to high-volume centers for pancreatectomy". *Annals of Surgical Oncology*. doi: 10.1245/s10434-022-13032-8.
Winchester, M. & B. King 2018. "Decentralization, healthcare access, and inequality in Mpumalanga, South Africa". *Health & Place* 51: 200–207.
World Health Organization 2019. *WHO Global Report on Traditional and Complementary Medicine*. Geneva. https://iris.who.int/items/0dc0d605-b1c3-4350-b62e-984b47688442.
World Health Organization 2024. Global Spending on Health: Emerging from the Pandemic. https://iris.who.int/handle/10665/379750.
Wright T. *et al.* 2021. "Accessing and utilising gender-affirming healthcare in England and Wales: trans and non-binary people's accounts of navigating gender identity clinics". *BMC Health Services Research*. doi: 10.1186/s12913-021-06661-4.
Xu, R. *et al.* 2022. "Trends in the disparities and equity of the distribution of traditional Chinese medicine health resources in China from 2010 to 2020". *PLOS One*, doi: 10.1371/journal.pone.0275712.
Yan, X. & S. He 2020. "The co-evolution of therapeutic landscape and health tourism in Bama longevity villages, China: an actor-network perspective". *Health & Place* 66. doi: 10.1016/j.healthplace.2020.102448.
Yee, R. *et al.* 2024. "COVID-19 vaccination site accessibility, United States, December 11, 2020–March 29, 2022". *Emerging Infectious Diseases* 30. doi: 10.3201/eid3005.230357.
Yee, V. *et al.* 2022. "Paradox of telemedicine: building or neglecting trust and equity". *Lancet Digital Health*. doi: 10.1016/S2589-7500(22)00100-5.
Yilma, M. *et al.* 2023. "Geographic disparities in access to liver transplantation". *Liver Transplantation*. doi: 10.1097/LVT.0000000000000182.
Young, T. *et al.* 2016. "Healthcare in Canada's North: are we getting value for money?" *Healthcare Policy* 12(1): 59–70.
Yu, E. & H. Amri 2016. "China's other medical systems: recognizing Uyghur, Tibetan, and Mongolian traditional medicines". *Global Advances in Health & Medicine* 5. doi: 10.7453/gahmj.2015.116.
Yu, H. *et al.* 2021. "Equity analysis of Chinese physician allocation based on Gini coefficient and Theil index". *BMC Health Services Research*. doi: 10.1186/s12913-021-06348-w.
Yu, L. *et al.* 2024. "Using smartphone user mobility to unveil actual travel time to healthcare: an example of mental health facilities". *Health & Place*. doi: 10.1016/j.healthplace.2024.103375.
Yu, S. *et al.* 2017. "The scope and impact of mobile health clinics in the United States: a literature review". *International Journal for Equity in Health*. doi: 10.1186/s12939-017-0671-2.
Zavras, D. *et al.* 2016. "Economic crisis, austerity and unmet healthcare needs: the case of Greece". *BMC Health Services Research*. doi: 10.1186/s12913-016-1557-5.
Zhang, J. *et al.* 2023. "Quantifying digital health inequality across a national healthcare system". *BMJ Health & Care Informatics*. doi: 10.1136/ bmjhci-2023-100809.
Zhang, X. *et al.* 2017. "Urban–rural differences in the association between access to healthcare and health outcomes among older adults in China". *BMC Geriatrics*. doi: 10.1186/s12877-017-0538-9.

INDEX

EU Authorised Representative:
Easy Access System Europe Mustamäe tee 50, 10621 Tallinn, Estonia
gpsr.requests@easproject.com

Printed and bound by CPI Group (UK) Ltd, Croydon, CR0 4YY
25/08/2026
02203506-0002